# The Practical CBT + DBT + ACT Workbook (10 in 1)

*250+ Cognitive Behavioral Therapy + Dialectical Behavior Therapy + Acceptance & Commitment Therapy + Vagus Nerve, Somatic Exercises and Tools for Beginners*

### Andrew C Hinkelberg

# © Copyright 2024. Andrew C Hinkelberg. All rights reserved.

The content contained within this book may not be reproduced, duplicated, or transmitted without direct written permission from the author or the publisher.

Under no circumstances will any blame or legal responsibility be held against the publisher or author for any damages, reparation, or monetary loss due to the information contained within this book, either directly or indirectly.

Legal Notice:

This book is copyright-protected. It is only for personal use. You cannot amend, distribute, sell, use, quote, or paraphrase any part of the content within this book without the consent of the author or publisher.

Disclaimer Notice:

Please note the information contained within this document is for educational and entertainment purposes only. All efforts have been executed to present accurate, up-to- date, reliable, and complete information. No warranties of any kind are declared or implied. Readers acknowledge that the author is not engaged in the rendering of legal, financial, medical, or professional advice. The content within this book has been derived from various sources. Please consult a licensed professional before attempting any techniques outlined in this book.

By reading this document, the reader agrees that under no circumstances is the author responsible for any losses, direct or indirect, that are incurred as a result of the use of the information contained within this document, including, but not limited to, errors, omissions, or inaccuracies.

# Table of Contents

Introduction .................................................................................................................................. 8
Chapter 1: Introduction to Cognitive Behavioral Therapy ............................................. 11
    History and Development of CBT ................................................................................... 11
    Core Principles of CBT ....................................................................................................... 13
    Identifying Distortions in Thinking .................................................................................. 15
        How to Prevent Distortive Thinking .......................................................................... 16
        Exercise to Identify Your Distorted Thoughts ........................................................ 18
    Cognitive Restructuring Techniques ............................................................................. 20
        Challenging Negative Thoughts ............................................................................... 21
        Positive Affirmations ................................................................................................... 21
        Visualization Techniques ............................................................................................ 22
        Behavioral Experiments ............................................................................................. 23
    Fundamental and Foundational CBT Exercises ........................................................ 23
        Positive Affirmations Exercise ................................................................................... 26
        Guided Meditation Exercise ..................................................................................... 27
    Concluding Thoughts ........................................................................................................ 28
Chapter 2: Techniques and Tools of Cognitive Behavioral Therapy ........................... 30
    Behavioral Activation ...................................................................................................... 30
    Thought Records and Journaling .................................................................................. 33
        Thought Journaling Exercise ..................................................................................... 36
    Exposure Therapy Guidelines ......................................................................................... 37
        Journaling Your Exposure Therapy .......................................................................... 41
    CBT for Anxiety Management ....................................................................................... 45
        Role-Playing Exercise ................................................................................................. 47
    Personalized CBT Action Plans ....................................................................................... 49
        Personalized Plans Encourage Accountability and Targeted Action ............ 49

    SMART Goals Lend Structure and Purpose ................................................................... 50
    Regular Check-Ins for Reevaluation and Celebration ................................................ 51
    Supplementing Personal Efforts with External Resources ...................................... 51
  Journaling Prompts ............................................................................................................................ 52
  Summary and Reflections of CBT Techniques and Tools ................................................. 54

## Chapter 3: Introduction to Dialectical Behavior Therapy ............................................. 57

  Origins and Theoretical Foundations of DBT ......................................................................... 57
  Four Modules of DBT Skills ............................................................................................................ 59
    Mindfulness ....................................................................................................................................... 59
    Distress Tolerance ......................................................................................................................... 60
    Emotional Regulation .................................................................................................................. 61
    Interpersonal Effectiveness ...................................................................................................... 61
  Self-Awareness and Mindfulness in DBT .................................................................................. 62
  Distress Tolerance Strategies ....................................................................................................... 64
  DBT's Approach to Emotional Regulation .............................................................................. 67
  Journaling Prompts ............................................................................................................................ 68
  Bringing It All Together With DBT ................................................................................................ 72

## Chapter 4: Practicing DBT Skills ............................................................................................... 73

  Interpersonal Effectiveness Roles ................................................................................................ 74
  DBT Diary Cards .................................................................................................................................. 78
    Why Use Diary Cards? ................................................................................................................. 78
    How to Use Diary Cards Successfully ................................................................................. 79
  Crisis Survival Techniques ............................................................................................................. 80
  Validation and Self-Soothing Practices .................................................................................... 82
    The Concept of Validation ........................................................................................................ 82
    Practicing Self-Validation .......................................................................................................... 83
    Developing Self-Soothing Strategies ................................................................................... 83
  Skills for Balancing Acceptance and Change ....................................................................... 84
  Journaling Prompts ............................................................................................................................ 86
  Final Thoughts on Practicing DBT Skills .................................................................................. 92

## Chapter 5: Introduction to Acceptance and Commitment Therapy ....................... 93

  Principles of Psychological Flexibility ....................................................................................... 94
  Understanding and Practicing Acceptance .......................................................................... 96

- Naming Your Discomfort ........................................................................... 98
- Role of Mindfulness in ACT ....................................................................... 99
  - Journaling Prompts That Inspire Mindfulness ................................... 101
- Values-Driven Life Planning ..................................................................... 105
- Journaling Prompts .................................................................................... 107
- Final Thoughts on ACT as a Practice ...................................................... 112

## Chapter 6: Applying ACT Techniques ........................................................ 113
- Everyday Mindfulness Exercises ............................................................... 114
  - Mindful Breathing ................................................................................. 114
  - Body Scan Meditation .......................................................................... 115
  - Mindful Eating ....................................................................................... 115
  - Walking Meditation ............................................................................... 116
- Identifying and Developing Your Values .................................................. 118
  - Values Exploration Exercise ................................................................. 118
  - Values Hierarchy Creation .................................................................... 119
  - Vision Board Activity ............................................................................. 119
  - Check-In Process .................................................................................. 120
  - Values Journaling Prompts .................................................................. 120
- Acceptance and Willingness Exercises ................................................... 126
  - Acceptance Journaling Exercise ......................................................... 126
  - Willingness Practice .............................................................................. 127
  - Visualization Techniques ...................................................................... 127
  - Surrender Demonstration ..................................................................... 128
- Cognitive Defusion Exercises .................................................................... 128
- Committed Action Plans ............................................................................ 130
- Journaling Prompts .................................................................................... 131
- Final Thoughts on ACT Techniques ......................................................... 135

## Chapter 7: Understanding the Vagus Nerve ............................................. 137
- The Anatomy and Functioning of the Vagus Nerve .............................. 138
- Polyvagal Theory Basics ............................................................................ 139
  - Understanding Neuroception ............................................................. 139
  - Considering Mobilization ..................................................................... 140
  - Its Role in Emotional Health ................................................................ 141

| | |
|---|---|
| Vagus Nerve Stimulation Practices | 142 |
| How to Take Your Vagus Nerve Health to the Next Level | 143 |
| Loving-Kindness Meditation | 145 |
| Breathing Exercises to Activate the Vagus Nerve | 148 |
| Impacts on Stress and Relaxation Responses | 151 |
| Journaling Prompts | 153 |
| Final Insights on the Vagus Nerve | 156 |
| **Chapter 8: Somatic Practices for Emotional Well-Being** | **158** |
| Basics of SE | 159 |
| SE: Understanding the Body's Role in Healing | 159 |
| Tracking and Grounding Practices | 161 |
| Body Scans and PMR | 163 |
| Movement-Based Therapies and Exercises | 166 |
| Connection Between Body and Mind Awareness | 170 |
| The Interconnectedness of Thoughts, Emotions, and Physical Sensations | 170 |
| Daily Practices and Feedback Loops | 171 |
| Addressing the Disconnection Brought on by Stress | 171 |
| Advocacy for Continued Practice of Body Awareness | 172 |
| Journal Prompts | 173 |
| Closing Remarks on Somatic Practices | 176 |
| **Chapter 9: Eye Movement Desensitization and Reprocessing** | **177** |
| Overview of EMDR Methodology | 178 |
| Phases of EMDR Treatment | 181 |
| Phase 1: History Taking and Treatment Planning | 181 |
| Phase 2: The Preparation Phase | 181 |
| Phase 3: The Assessment Phase | 181 |
| Phase 4: The Desensitization Phase | 182 |
| Phase 5: The Installation Phase | 182 |
| Phase 6: The Body Scan Phase | 182 |
| Phase 7: Closure | 182 |
| Phase 8: The Reevaluation Phase | 183 |
| Journaling for EMDR Processing | 183 |
| Enhancing EMDR Effectiveness with Journaling | 183 |

- Specific Journaling Prompts Tailored for EMDR Work ........ 184
  - Alignment with EMDR's Phases ........ 185
  - Long-Term Benefits of Regular EMDR-Focused Journaling ........ 185
- Self-Administered EMDR Techniques ........ 186
  - Visualizing for EMDR ........ 188
- Journaling Prompts ........ 191
- Final Thoughts on EMDR ........ 194

## Chapter 10: Integrative Approaches for Holistic Healing ........ 195
- Creating a Personalized Mental Health Toolkit ........ 196
  - Self-Reflection Journal Prompts ........ 199
- Daily Routines for Sustained Emotional Resilience ........ 206
  - *Establishing Morning Rituals* ........ *206*
  - *Incorporating Mindfulness Breaks* ........ *206*
  - *Evening Reflection Practices* ........ *207*
  - *Consistency and Adjustment* ........ *207*
  - *Practical Guidelines for Implementation* ........ *207*
- Building Support Systems and Resources ........ 209
- Evaluating Progress and Adjusting Strategies ........ 212
- Long-Term Commitment to Mental Health ........ 213
- Evening Reflections ........ 215
- Concluding Thoughts ........ 220

## Conclusion ........ 221
## Glossary ........ 225
## References ........ 228

# Introduction

Have you ever felt trapped by your thoughts, struggling to escape patterns that repeat endlessly? What if you had a set of practical tools right at your fingertips that helped you break free and lead the fulfilling life you've always dreamed of?

Many of us find ourselves caught in cycles of anxiety, depression, or emotional turmoil, which can be extremely overwhelming. Our minds can be our worst enemies as we focus on our adverse circumstances and critique ourselves more than anyone else. But what if it didn't have to be this way? What if there were concrete steps you could take, starting today, to unravel these mental constraints and reclaim control over your mental and emotional well-being?

This book is designed to guide you through over 250 actionable therapy prompts and exercises—strategies that can empower you to take charge of your mental well-being regardless of what's occurring in your life. Whether you struggle with mental health challenges or seek self-improvement, or you are a mental health practitioner looking for practical tools for your clients, this book offers invaluable resources you can use and modify to meet your needs.

You might wonder how one book can cater to such diverse needs. The answer lies in the diversity of the therapeutic approaches covered within these pages. From the structured frameworks of cognitive behavioral therapy (CBT) to the mindful practices of acceptance and commitment therapy (ACT), each chapter unveils unique skills and exercises to enrich your journey of self-development. You may even connect deeply with the goal-setting techniques in solution-focused brief therapy, or the expressive outlets provided through art therapy. There is no one-size-fits-all solution to mental health, so a broad spectrum of methods is valuable in finding a strategy that resonates with you most.

With the knowledge you gain throughout this book, you will start viewing setbacks as steppingstones that help you grow. Discovering resilience and inner peace during turbulent times can make navigating them more accessible. Through real-life stories and examples, you will learn how many others have walked difficult paths and come out stronger and happier. By practicing the various journaling prompts and mindfulness exercises throughout this book, you can be inspired to embrace your inner strength for lasting growth.

Change isn't passive; it demands active participation. By committing to the exercises outlined in this book, you're not just reading about transformation—you're practicing it. It's essential to remember that while knowledge is power, action is what sets change in motion. Each prompt or exercise is a step forward, a brick laid down on the path to a healthier, more balanced life. It takes courage to face your struggles and dedication to work through them consistently. But with persistence, you will see progress, however gradual.

Before starting this book, take a moment to reflect on what brought you here. What are you hoping to achieve? What aspects of your life do you want to enhance or change entirely? Keeping these questions in mind will help you stay focused and motivated as you encounter the ups and downs of this journey. Remember, it's okay to start small. If anything, it's the best approach to take. Small steps can lead to significant strides over time. Begin with the exercises that feel most accessible to you, and as you become more comfortable, challenge yourself to tackle the more complex ones. By doing this, you will work at your own pace and eventually develop various skills that keep you emotionally balanced.

One of the most empowering aspects of this journey is the realization that you can influence your mental state and emotional responses. Although it can be challenging, you are in the driver's seat. This book encourages you to take ownership of your mental health, providing you with the resources and guidance to become your support system. This doesn't mean you must do it alone; support from friends, family, or a professional can be invaluable. However, knowing you have the tools to manage your mental well- being on your terms can also be incredibly liberating.

The journey toward better mental health and personal growth is ongoing and ever- evolving. It requires patience, effort, and a willingness to embrace the process. But rest assured: Every step you take brings you closer to a place of greater understanding, balance, and fulfillment. Use this book as your companion on that journey, offering guidance, encouragement, and practical tools to help you navigate the ups and downs.

Are you ready to take control of your emotional well-being? With an open heart and a committed spirit, you have the potential to create meaningful, lasting change in your life. Let this book guide you as you explore new ways of thinking, feeling, and being. The path to mental well-being and personal growth is not always easy, but it is undoubtedly worth taking. Welcome to the first step of a rewarding adventure!

# Chapter 1: Introduction to Cognitive Behavioral Therapy

The first therapy strategy we'll be discussing can help you manage a wide array of emotional challenges. Cognitive behavioral therapy (CBT) has been a pillar in the field of mental health for years, and it's a practice that can be explored on your own at home. CBT is a structured approach that focuses on changing unhelpful thought patterns and behaviors to prevent feelings of anxiety, depression, and other emotional difficulties. This chapter unpacks CBT's foundational concepts, helping you identify how cognitive practices can significantly improve your emotional well-being.

Let's journey through the origins of CBT, tracing its development from the pioneering work of Aaron Beck and Albert Ellis to its current status as an evidence-based therapeutic practice. This chapter will teach you about the core principles of CBT, such as recognizing cognitive distortions and employing Socratic questioning and behavioral activation. You'll also receive practical exercises for beginners, allowing you to apply CBT techniques daily. Whether you want to enhance your mental health, support others in their emotional journeys, or enrich your professional knowledge, this exploration into CBT will be invaluable.

## History and Development of CBT

As one of the most influential and widely recognized forms of psychotherapy, CBT helps countless individuals manage and overcome mental health issues. To truly understand its impact, it's essential to learn about its evolution—from its roots in the 1960s to its current standing as a cornerstone of psychological treatment.

CBT emerged during an era when traditional psychoanalytic methods dominated the field. In contrast to these approaches, which often focus primarily on patients' unconscious motivations and early life experiences, CBT concentrates on the here and now. This new methodology was grounded in scientific research and aimed to create evidence-based practices that could be systematically evaluated for effectiveness. The shift toward a more factual approach significantly departed from earlier therapeutic paradigms.

The development of CBT owes much to the pioneering work of Aaron Beck and Albert Ellis. Both clinicians were dissatisfied with the results of traditional psychoanalysis despite their extensive training and expertise in those areas. Beck, initially trained as a psychiatrist, began observing patterns in his patients' thought processes and noticed that depressive symptoms often accompanied negative thought patterns. He theorized that these cognitive distortions were not merely symptoms but pivotal emotional distress causes. Based on this insight, Beck developed cognitive therapy, the precursor to modern-day CBT, which emphasizes identifying and restructuring dysfunctional thoughts to improve emotional well-being (Beck, 2019).

Albert Ellis contributed significantly to the development of rational emotive behavior therapy, another foundation of CBT. Ellis proposed that irrational beliefs and unrealistic expectations underlie many emotional problems. He found that we can significantly alleviate our emotional distress by challenging and replacing these irrational beliefs with more rational ones. The work of both Beck and Ellis highlighted the central role of cognition in mental health, setting the stage for the broader acceptance and application of CBT.

Over the past decades, research has consistently validated CBT's effectiveness across various conditions. Numerous studies have demonstrated marked improvements in anxiety, depression, post-traumatic stress disorder, obsessive-compulsive disorder, and many other mental health issues through the use of CBT techniques. Randomized controlled trials, the gold standard in clinical research, have repeatedly shown that CBT can substantially reduce symptoms and long-lasting improvements in well-being (Beck et al., 2020).

Digital and online delivery methods have also expanded the reach of CBT. Online platforms, apps, and teletherapy provide additional avenues for us to access CBT, making it possible for people in remote or underserved areas to receive high-quality psychological care. These digital solutions not only enhance accessibility but also cater to modern lifestyles, offering flexibility and convenience without compromising the effectiveness of treatment.

CBT has evolved dramatically since its inception and integrates well with other therapeutic techniques. For instance, combining CBT with medication management, mindfulness techniques, or other behavioral therapies can enhance overall treatment outcomes. This integrative approach allows for a more comprehensive management of mental health challenges.

## Core Principles of CBT

CBT is a widely known and appreciated therapeutic technique for addressing various mental health issues, including anxiety, depression, and emotional regulation. The fundamental concepts of this practice showcase how effective it is for improving your mental health. Here are some core principles to consider:

- **Understanding cognitive distortions.** One of CBT's core principles is identifying and understanding cognitive distortions. Cognitive distortions are common thinking errors that impact your emotions and behavior. These irrational or exaggerated thoughts can lead to negative feelings and actions. Recognizing these distortions is crucial for identifying negative thought patterns that are often untrue. Examples of cognitive distortions include all-or-nothing thinking, overgeneralization, and catastrophizing, which will be explored in greater detail shortly. By becoming aware of these errors, you can challenge and change your harmful beliefs, improving your emotional well-being.

- **Practicing behavioral activation.** Behavioral activation is another crucial concept in CBT. This technique emphasizes taking action to counter negative thoughts and emotions. The idea is that practicing positive activities can break the cycle of negative thinking and feelings. Behavioral activation emphasizes the interconnection between thoughts, feelings, and behavior. For instance, if you're experiencing depression, you may withdraw from social activities, which, in turn, intensifies your negative thoughts and feelings. Encouraging proactive engagement in enjoyable and meaningful activities elevates your mood and provides emotional relief when faced with stressful times.

- **Using Socratic questioning.** Socratic questioning is a method used in CBT to challenge and restructure negative thoughts. This technique involves asking a series of guided questions to help you examine the validity of your thoughts and develop new perspectives through self-reflection. Socratic questioning influences critical thinking and enables you to identify irrational thoughts and replace them with more realistic and balanced ones. Examples of Socratic questions include "What evidence do I have to support this thought?" "Is there an alternative explanation?" and "What would I tell a friend in a similar situation?" Answering these questions helps you identify valuable information about your thought patterns to begin adopting healthier ways of thinking.

- **Working from home.** CBT is a practice that's easily accessible because it can be done at home. These exercises don't have to be practiced in therapy, as you can track your thoughts and behaviors independently. Such homework may entail keeping a thought record and documenting negative thoughts and the situations that trigger them. This allows for greater awareness and opportunitiesto practice cognitive restructuring techniques. You reinforce your learning by consistently completing homework assignments, making applying CBT principles in your everyday life easier. These exercises also encourage ongoing self- reflection and accountability, which are essential for long-term success in mental health management.

All these elements of CBT will be explored in more detail throughout the book. By understanding your cognitive process first, you'll be able to navigate CBT at home in a way that's suited to your needs. You can make the most of your CBT journey through techniques such as behavioral activations, Socratic questioning, and many others explored in the following two chapters.

## Identifying Distortions in Thinking

Identifying and analyzing cognitive distortions is a crucial part of CBT. These distortions are irrational or exaggerated thought patterns that reinforce negative thinking and emotions. Recognizing distortive thinking can often be challenging because you grow accustomed to this pessimistic mindset. Here are some common types of distortive thinking:

- **All-or-nothing thinking.** One of the most common cognitive distortions is all- or-nothing thinking, also known as "black-and-white thinking." If you practice this thinking, you view situations in absolute terms, meaning everything is good or bad, successful or failed, with no middle ground. This thinking can lead to extreme reactions and intense stress when outcomes do not align perfectly with your expectations. For instance, a student who receives a B on a test may feel like a complete failure because they did not get an A, disregarding the positive aspects of their performance.

- **Overgeneralization.** Overgeneralization is another prevalent negative thought process. In this pattern, a single adverse event is viewed as part of a never-ending pattern of defeat. If you engage in such thinking, you might use such words as "always" or "never" to describe situations, leading to feelings of hopelessness. An example would be someone who concludes that they will never find employment after one unsuccessful job interview and that future efforts are pointless.

- **Catastrophic thinking.** Catastrophizing involves anticipating the worst possible outcome in any given situation, often without considering more likely and realistic results. This distortion amplifies anxiety and fear, making problems seem insurmountable. For example, if someone makes a minor mistake at work, they might fear being fired or facing severe reprimands, even though such extreme consequences are unlikely.

### How to Prevent Distortive Thinking

Recognizing patterns in your thinking is crucial when addressing these distortions. When you're aware of these thought processes, you can analyze and transform them into more productive and positive thoughts.

The following strategies can make it easier for you to prevent distortive thinking:

- **Self-assessment exercises.** Self-assessment exercises such as journaling can be highly effective in healing distortive thinking. By maintaining a journal, you can track recurring cognitive distortions over time, noting specific instances when you've engaged in distorted thinking. This practice helps you identify patterns and triggers contributing to negative thoughts and clarifies how these distortions affect daily life.

- **Distortion exercises.** Distortion exercises serve as another valuable tool for documenting and analyzing specific thoughts. These activities help you categorize thoughts to identify underlying cognitive errors and provide structured ways to challenge and reframe them. For instance, recording automatic thoughts is a widely used CBT tool that prompts you to document automatic negative thoughts, assess their emotional impact, and develop more adaptive responses. This method highlights the presence of distortions and encourages critical thinking and proactive problem-solving.

- **Real-life applications.** Applying real-life examples in daily scenarios can further enhance your ability to identify and manage cognitive distortions. Practicing this skill consistently leads to better emotional regulation and greater overall resilience. For instance, if you frequently experience social anxiety and tend to catastrophize social interactions, actively challenging your distortive thoughts during a conversation or while preparing for a social event can gradually reduce anxiety and build confidence. Real-life practice is essential for the successful implementation of these techniques. Incorporating cognitive restructuring into daily activities, such as during stressful situations at work or conflicts in personal relationships, reinforces the skills learned through CBT exercises. Continuous application helps solidify new thought patterns, making your thoughts more intuitive and less distortive.

- **Distortive thinking**. In addition to personal practices, training yourself to identify cognitive distortions in others can also help.

Engaging in supportive dialogue with friends or family members about their thought patterns can influence mutual understanding and strengthen your bonds. Noticing when loved ones exhibit all-or-nothing thinking, overgeneralization, or catastrophizing allows for compassionate interventions and shared learning opportunities.

- **Cognitive restructuring techniques.** These techniques complement the identification process by offering strategies to challenge and change distorted thoughts. Here, techniques such as Socratic questioning can help you test the validity of negative beliefs, encouraging you to consider alternative and more realistic perspectives. Questions such as "What evidence do I have for this thought?" or "Is there another way to look at this situation?" promote critical analysis and facilitate the development of balanced, rational thinking.

As you practice these tips, remember that supportive environments also play a vital role in this journey. Communities, whether online or offline, that focus on mental health and self-improvement can offer encouragement and shared experiences. Participating in group discussions or therapy sessions allows you to learn from others' experiences, gain new insights, and receive feedback on your progress.

### Exercise to Identify Your Distorted Thoughts

The following exercise can help you identify and process the negative thoughts holding you back mentally and emotionally. Answer the following multiple-choice questions to determine which type of distortive thinking you practice:

## Choose the statement that best reflects your thought pattern in a challenging situation:

- "I always mess things up."
- "I might not do well, but I can learn from the experience."
- "There's no way I can succeed."

## When you receive feedback, how do you typically react?
- "That just proves I'm not good enough."
- "I can use this to improve next time."
- "It's not worth listening to; they don't understand my situation."

## How do you view your accomplishments?
- "They don't matter because I could have done better."
- "I'm proud of what I achieved despite the challenges."
- "I was just lucky this time."

## In a social situation, what thoughts do you have?
- "I'll embarrass myself."
- "I enjoy connecting with others."
- "I don't belong here."

## What do you think about the future?
- "It's going to be terrible."
- "I can find ways to make it better."
- "I have no control over it."

## When faced with a problem, what is your usual response?
- "I can't handle this."
- "I'll break it down and tackle it step by step."
- "There's no point in even trying."

## How do you feel about conflicts with others?

- "They always end badly."

- "I can communicate and work through issues."
- "It's easier just to ignore the problem."

**When comparing yourself to others, what do you often think?**
- "I'll never measure up."
- "Everyone has their strengths and weaknesses."
- "I am only a failure."

**If you make a mistake, how do you interpret it?**
- "That proves I'm a failure."
- "Mistakes are part of learning."
- "I should just give up."

**Reflecting on your life, what sticks out to you?**
- "All the ways I haven't succeeded."
- "The growth I've experienced over time."
- "I haven't done anything worthwhile."

After you have completed this exercise, reflect on your answers. Look for patterns that indicate a tendency toward cognitive distortions. If you mostly picked A or C, it's a sign that you often experience distorted thoughts. However, if you mostly picked B's, it's a sign that you have more realistic thought processes. Think about how these thoughts impact your mood and behaviors. Consider how you can challenge these thoughts in your daily life. An excellent way to start is to write down a common negative thought and list evidence that contradicts that thought. This can help you see things from a different perspective.

## Cognitive Restructuring Techniques

When discussing restructuring cognitive distortions in CBT, we emphasize the importance of transforming productive thought patterns. These shifts can significantly improve how you feel and behave daily.

Let's explore the methods used to achieve this mental transformation.

## Challenging Negative Thoughts

You must first challenge the negative thoughts you identify to change your thought patterns. This process involves identifying distorted beliefs and questioning their accuracy instead of accepting them as genuine. For instance, if you frequently think, "I always fail at everything I do," it's essential to pause and examine this thought critically. Ask yourself: What evidence supports this belief? What evidence contradicts it?

Constructing counterstatements is another powerful technique for invalidating negative thoughts. If you think, "I'll never be good enough," replace it with a more balanced statement like, "I am still learning and growing, and that's okay." These counterstatements are positive spins and honest reflections that reduce distortive

thinking. Repeating and consistently practicing this can reshape your cognitive framework to be more constructive and empowering.

Keeping a journal where you document these negative thoughts, and the corresponding counterstatements is helpful. This practice can make it easier to track progress and reinforce positive changes. Over time, the goal is to see fewer documents of negative thoughts in your journal, showcasing that the CBT is working.

## Positive Affirmations

While you reframe these negative absolute thoughts into something more realistic, you can utilize positive affirmations. Positive affirmations are personalized statements designed to foster a more optimistic self-image. These should be specific and meaningful to you. For example, if you struggle with self-esteem, an affirmation could be, "I am worthy of love and respect."

Creating a daily routine for reciting these affirmations can be particularly effective. This habit slowly rewires your brain to focus on strengths and potential rather than weaknesses and failures. Repeating your affirmations helps reinforce your positive beliefs in your subconscious mind, which gradually influences your automatic thoughts.

Write down your affirmations and place them where you will see them frequently—on your bathroom mirror or desk or make it the screensaver on your phone or computer. The constant visual cues help reinforce these positive thoughts throughout your day. At the end of this chapter, you will find an affirmations activity that can help you use this practice successfully.

## *Visualization Techniques*

Visualization is a mental imagery exercise that replaces negative beliefs with positive outcomes. This technique is a form of mental transformation, as you focus on a more favorable result that may not be your current reality.

Suppose you have an important presentation coming up and are overwhelmed by thoughts of failure. In that case, visualization can help you vividly imagine yourself delivering the presentation confidently and effectively and receiving positive feedback from your audience. This can reduce anxiety, promote self-belief, and even manifest a positive performance.

Guided exercises can facilitate this process. Often, scripts are available to help you imagine yourself residing in a safe space or achieving a particular goal. Practicing these guided visualizations regularly can build confidence and reduce anxiety linked to specific situations.

Set aside a few minutes each day for visualization exercises. Find a quiet space, close your eyes, and immerse yourself fully in the cheerful scene you want to create. To practice guided visualizations successfully, use the exercise at the end of this chapter.

## *Behavioral Experiments*

Behavioral experiments are achieved by testing the validity of your beliefs through real- world actions. This practical approach allows you to confront and evaluate the outcomes of your thoughts and predictions. For example, if you believe that people will reject you if you speak up in a group, a behavioral experiment might involve participating actively in a meeting and observing the reactions. You will likely find that everyone receives you well and that it's not as scary as you thought.

Engaging in these experiments might seem daunting, but the confidence you gain afterward can be liberating. Often, you'll find that your fears and pessimistic predictions are exaggerated and much worse than reality. You will develop a more realistic and positive outlook on life by consistently testing these negative beliefs.

Before engaging in a behavioral experiment, write your expectations and fears about the outcome in your journal. Afterward, note what happened and compare the two. This reflective practice reinforces the lessons learned and encourages continued experimentation.

# Fundamental and Foundational CBT Exercises

Before we walk through some specific CBT exercises in the next chapter, let's focus on some fundamental and foundational activities to get you started with this practice. These exercises are designed to help manage anxiety and depression and improve overall emotional regulation. The following points discuss these exercises on the surface level. In the next chapter, you will find specific exercises for each point:

- **Thought records.** Let's start with thought records, essential tools for tracking negative and positive thoughts. Thought records encourage self-exploration by providing a structured method to analyze your daily events and responses. When you document your thoughts in real time, it becomes easier to identify patterns and understand how specific thoughts affect your emotions and behavior. For example, if you find yourself feeling anxious before social events, recording the particular thoughts contributing to your anxiety allows you to dissect them. You might write down, "I feel like I might say something embarrassing," and then challenge this thought by recalling past social events where things went smoothly. This regular practice influences you to prioritize positive thinking. The more you practice thought records, the better your thinking patterns will become. We'll discuss the practice of thought records in greater detail in upcoming chapters.

- **Behavioral activation.** Next, let's consider behavioral activation. This practice is designed to guide you through engaging in activities that can lift your mood and promote emotional well-being. When you feel depressed, you may find that the idea of being active can seem overwhelming. However, breaking tasks into manageable chunks using these activities and worksheets can make it more manageable. One practical approach is to create an activity schedule, which involves dividing each day into one-hour blocks and planning specific activities for each block. This structure helps regulate daily routines, such as sleeping and eating patterns and encourages a gradual reengagement in hobbies or social activities you've been avoiding. For instance, scheduling a simple walk in the park or a brief phone call with a friend can be a practical step toward improving your mood (Swainston, 2021).

- **Goal setting.** Goal setting is another critical component of CBT. As always, it's valuable to prioritize setting SMART—Specific, Measurable, Attainable, Realistic, and Time-bound—goals.

Establishing SMART goals helps break down more extensive, often overwhelming, objectives into smaller, more achievable steps. This process can inspire motivation and give you a sense of direction. Suppose that your ultimate goal is to reduce your anxiety in social settings. In that case, a SMART goal might be attending one social event weekly for a month, gradually increasing your comfort level. Another example might be aiming to complete a specific project at work within a set timeframe, helping you build confidence through your gradual successes. Setting these detailed milestones gives you a more straightforward path and makes it easier to track your progress and adjust as needed.

- **Reflective journaling.** Reflection prompts are equally valuable for maintaining ongoing self-awareness. Journaling regularly about your thoughts, feelings, and experiences allows you to reflect on your progress and remain engaged with CBT practices. Reflection prompts can serve as a guide for what to write about. For example, you might start with questions like, "What was a challenging moment for me today, and how did I handle it?" or "What positive interaction did I have, and what can I learn from it?" This reflection routine facilitates a deeper understanding of your experiences and the development of new coping strategies. Over time, these journal entries can become a powerful record of your growth, showcasing the hurdles you've overcome and the strides you've made in your mental health journey. Throughout the various chapters, you will receive reflective prompts to help your journal.

- **Be consistent.** As with any changes you make in life, consistency is essential to reap accurate results. Incorporating these fundamental CBT exercises into your daily routine can yield significant benefits. Thought records allow for a structured exploration of your internal dialogue, while behavioral activation exercises provide a roadmap to proactive emotional engagement.

Goal setting,

- mainly through the SMART framework, ensures your aspirations are clear and attainable. Reflective journaling deepens your self-awareness and keeps you connected to the therapeutic process.

By integrating these tools, you can develop an effective system and routine for managing your anxiety, depression, and other emotional challenges. Each exercise complements the others, creating a comprehensive approach to fostering better mental health. Thought records delve into cognitive patterns, behavioral activation promotes action, goal setting provides direction, and reflection prompts ensure engagement. As you adopt these practices, their cumulative effects can substantially improve your overall well-being.

### Positive Affirmations Exercise

Practicing positive affirmations is a simple and effective way to transform your thoughts. Continuously empowering your mind with positive thoughts can give you a more optimistic mindset. Here are some examples of positive affirmations:

- I believe in my abilities and strengths.
- I am worthy of love and respect.
- I embrace challenges as opportunities for growth.
- My potential is limitless, and I can achieve my goals.
- I am surrounded by support and positive energy.
- I accept myself unconditionally and recognize my unique qualities.
- I attract abundance and success into my life.
- I am grateful for the opportunities that come my way.
- Each day, I grow stronger and more confident.
- I choose to focus on the good in every situation.
- I am at peace with my past and excited for my future.
- My thoughts shape my reality, and I choose positivity.
- I inspire those around me with my positive attitude.
- I release negative thoughts and make room for positive ones.

- I am in control of my thoughts and emotions.
- I cherish every moment and live life to the fullest.
- I am enough just as I am. I believe in the power of my dreams and pursue them.
- Challenges are steppingstones to my success.
- I radiate positivity and attract joy into my life.
- I trust the process of life and my journey.
- I can overcome any obstacle that comes my way.
- I choose happiness and find joy in the small things.
- I am loved and appreciated for who I am.
- I deserve to have fulfilled relationships.
- Each day brings new opportunities, and I embrace them.
- I choose to let go of negativity and embrace positivity.

## *Guided Meditation Exercise*

Guided meditation is one of the best exercises for emotional regulation and stress management. The following exercise can help you practice structured meditation to identify your thought patterns and emotions:

1. Find a quiet space where you can sit comfortably. Close your eyes gently and take a slow, deep breath through your nose. Hold it for a moment. Now, exhale slowly through your mouth. Repeat this and let your body relax with each breath. Focus on your breathing. Feel the air enter your lungs and feel your chest rise and fall. With each breath, let go of any tension you are holding.

2. As you continue to breathe, bring your attention to your thoughts. Notice them as they come and go. Do not judge them. Just observe. If an idea seems strong, acknowledge it and let it drift away like a cloud in the sky. Imagine each thought as a leaf floating on a stream. Watch it move and disappear. Allow yourself to be present in this moment without the need to hold on to any thought.

3. Now, focus on your emotions. What are you feeling right now? Identify the emotion without labeling it as good or bad. Is it happiness, sadness, stress, or calm? Just notice where you feel that emotion in your body. Is it in your chest, your stomach, or maybe in your head? Breathe into that space. Imagine sending warmth and light to that area with every breath, easing discomfort.

4. Shift your attention back to your breath. Breathe deeply, feeling your body expand with air. Hold it for a moment. As you exhale, imagine letting go of any lingering emotions that do not serve you right now. Allow them to flow out with your breath. Each exhale releases tension and negativity, leaving you feeling lighter and more relaxed.

5. Now, visualize a safe place. This could be a beach, a forest, or any spot that brings you peace. Imagine the sights and sounds of this place. Feel the warmth of the sun or the cool breeze. Picture yourself in that setting, entirely at ease. Allow the tranquility of this place to envelop you. Let it fill your heart with comfort.

6. As you remain in this peaceful visual, you can also think about your intentions. What do you hope to achieve with this meditation? Is it clarity, calmness, or confidence? Repeat your intention quietly in your mind. Let it resonate within you. With each breath, reinforce your commitment to this intention.

## Concluding Thoughts

Throughout this chapter, we have delved into the foundational aspects of CBT. By tracing its origins and understanding the contributions of key figures such as Aaron Beck and Albert Ellis, you now know how CBT has evolved into a leading method for addressing various mental health conditions. We explored core principles such as identifying cognitive distortions, which are crucial in recognizing and correcting negative thought patterns.

As you reflect on the knowledge that you have gained, it's clear that CBT offers practical and evidence-based strategies that can drastically improve your mental well-being. Whether you deal with anxiety or depression or are simply seeking personal growth, these techniques provide actionable steps toward better emotional regulation. CBT's adaptability and accessibility make it a well-known and widely practiced form of therapy. Integrating CBT techniques into your daily life allows you to endure change and become the best version of yourself.

This chapter focused on learning more about CBT, its history, and its powerful impact on mental health. As we move on to the next chapter, you will find practical exercises that help you practice CBT independently.

# Chapter 2: Techniques and Tools of Cognitive Behavioral Therapy

Now that you know more about cognitive behavioral therapy (CBT) and how it works, you can explore some techniques and tools to help you put CBT into practice.

In this chapter, we'll discuss various practical methods designed to help you regulate your emotional responses, providing you with the skills to navigate life's challenges more easily. These tools are helpful approaches to the mental and emotional issues that have been controlling your life and the way that you react to it.

This chapter will provide strategies and exercises to enhance your journey toward better emotional health and management. From behavioral activation worksheets that encourage engagement in meaningful activities to thought records and journaling techniques that help identify and challenge negative thinking patterns, each tool is crafted to enhance self-awareness and emotional regulation. You'll also learn about exposure therapy that can help you confront your fears while using personalized CBT action plans to meet your specific needs. All these tools and techniques will help you manage your anxiety, depression, and other emotional challenges with more ease.

## Behavioral Activation

Behavioral activation is a core technique in CBT that focuses on engaging you in meaningful activities to improve mood and reduce anxiety. It is particularly effective in breaking the cycle of avoidance that often causes emotional distress. Engaging in enjoyable activities can create positive experiences that counteract negative emotions. Here's how behavioral activation in the form of activities and exercises can help you improve your mental and emotional health:

- **Disrupt avoidant behavior.** Practicing activities that you enjoy can disrupt the pattern of avoidance that contributes to worsening emotional states. When people with avoidant personalities feel depressed or anxious, they tend to withdraw from their usual activities and social interactions. This withdrawal can lead to increased feelings of isolation, which further deteriorates their mental state. Behavioral activation comes into play here, because it encourages you to reengage in activities you enjoy and find fulfilling. For instance, if you love to paint but you've stopped due to depression, you may find it valuable to set aside time to engage in this activity that used to make you happy. By pushing through the initial resistance and beginning the activity, you will experience an improvement in your mood. Even if this uplifting experience is temporary, it helps you escape your mental struggles briefly.

- **Schedule regular activities.** Regularly scheduling activities is crucial in developing a healthy routine, providing structure, and offering a sense of predictability during emotional distress. When you experience anxiety or depression, your daily routine can become erratic, contributing to feelings of chaos and helplessness. Creating a structured schedule with planned activities can help prevent this. For example, going on a daily walk at the same time each morning provides physical benefits and establishes a predictable routine that can bring comfort and stability. A consistent schedule ensures that you engage in activities likely to boost your mood rather than resisting the urge to avoid them.

- **Start small.** Starting with small, manageable steps is critical for success in behavioral activation. When you are struggling with significant emotional distress, the idea of engaging in even moderately challenging activities can seem overwhelming. Therefore, beginning with activities that require minimal effort yet offer a sense of accomplishment is essential. For instance, instead of aiming to complete an entire workout session, start with a short 5-minute walk. These small victories are crucial, because they build confidence and create momentum for tackling more challenging tasks in the future. As confidence grows, so can the complexity and duration of the activities. When engaging in behavioral activation, breaking down larger goals into smaller actionable steps is helpful. This approach makes daunting tasks feel more achievable. For example, if someone aims to enhance their physical fitness, the first step might be simply wearing gym clothes and stepping outside. The next step could be walking to the corner store. Gradually, these steps can lead to joining a fitness class or going for a run. Individuals can make steady progress without feeling overwhelmed by focusing on a tiny step at a time.
- **Be thoughtful with plans.** Behavioral activation requires thoughtful planning and execution. Choosing activities that align with your values and interests is essential to maximize engagement and enjoyment. If family is a central value, activities include spending quality time with loved ones. If health is a priority, incorporating exercise, healthy cooking, or other wellness activities would be beneficial. Linking activities to your deeply held values makes you more likely to find meaning and motivation in your actions, which, in turn, reinforces their positive impact on your emotional well-being.
- **Incentivize yourself.** Rewarding yourself for completing activities can also reinforce the habit of staying active. Positive reinforcement through incentives you value can take your

consistency to the next level. Some forms of positive reinforcement you can explore include treating yourself to your favorite snack, enjoying a relaxing bath, or simply acknowledging the achievement internally. Rewarding yourself helps you associate the completion of activities with positive feelings, making it more likely for you to engage in behaviors that benefit your emotional health.

Actions are often more potent than words. While journaling and reflecting on your progress with words can be essential and meaningful, you sometimes need to take action to see tangible results.

## Thought Records and Journaling

Thought records and journaling are potent tools in CBT that help you gain control over your negative thoughts, emotions, and patterns. It's an easy and accessible way to keep yourself accountable throughout this transformative journey.

Thought records are a practical method for keeping track of your negative thoughts. This systematic approach is done by documenting specific situations that trigger negative thoughts, automatic negative thoughts, and the accompanying emotional responses. For example, if you're in a social situation where you feel ignored, you might jot down the event, your thoughts ("They don't like me"), and your feelings (upset or anxious). This practice enables you to recognize recurring themes in your thought patterns that contribute to anxiety or depression.

One significant benefit of clearly laying out situations, thoughts, emotions, and alternative responses is its clarity. By objectively writing down these elements, you can distance yourself from your immediate emotional reactions and look at the situation more rationally. This structured approach facilitates cognitive restructuring, where people identify and challenge irrational or unhelpful thoughts. Once a negative thought is identified, alternative, more balanced thoughts can be introduced. For example, instead of thinking, "I'm useless at my job," you might reframe the thought to, "I'm still learning and improving every day."

Set specific times for reflection through journaling and embedding emotional processing into daily life. Just like any other habit, consistency is critical. Allocating a few minutes each day for journaling ensures that you take the time to reflect on your thoughts and feelings regularly. This routine can be particularly beneficial during stressful periods, allowing you to process emotions rather than let them accumulate unchecked immediately. Regular reflection enhances self-awareness and promotes the continuous practice of CBT techniques, leading to long-term improvements in emotional regulation.

Furthermore, engaging in thought records and journaling can significantly improve decision-making and problem-solving abilities. By analyzing past entries, you can learn from previous experiences, identifying what worked well and what didn't. This retrospective analysis enables you to make more informed decisions in future situations, fostering a sense of mastery and control over your life.

If you're dealing with anxiety, thought records can be instrumental. Reviewing recorded thoughts allows you to spot patterns of avoidance, which is a common coping mechanism for anxiety. For instance, you might notice you tend to avoid social gatherings due to fears of being judged. Recognizing this pattern is the first step toward addressing it. By gradually challenging the thoughts associated with avoidance and confronting the feared situations, you can reduce anxiety over time (Wilding, 2015).

Similarly, if you're experiencing depression, thought records can highlight behaviors that reinforce negative feelings. For example, staying in bed all day might initially seem like a way to cope with exhaustion, but it often leads to increased feelings of isolation and worthlessness. Identifying such behaviors and understanding their impact is crucial. By using thought records to challenge the assumptions behind these behaviors ("Resting will make me feel better"), you can adopt more proactive approaches, such as engaging in activities that provide a sense of accomplishment and connection.

Journaling also supports the process of setting and achieving personal goals. By clearly defining goals using a journal, you can create a roadmap for personal development. Whether improving social skills, managing stress better, or building confidence, having written goals keeps you accountable. Tracking progress toward these goals using a journal provides a tangible measure of success, encouraging continued effort and dedication.

Incorporating reflective questions into journaling can further deepen self-exploration. Questions such as "What did I learn from today?" or "How did I handle a challenging situation?" prompt individuals to think critically about their experiences. This type of reflection not only aids in emotional processing but also contributes to personal growth by fostering a mindset of continuous improvement.

Another advantage of journaling is its role in enhancing communication and relationships. By recording interactions and related emotions, you can identify patterns in how you relate to others.

For instance, specific topics of conversation frequently lead to misunderstandings or conflicts. Recognizing these patterns allows for more mindful communication in future interactions, improving relationship dynamics.

Tracking progress in therapy through journaling can also be highly beneficial. Sharing journal entries with a therapist provides valuable context for therapeutic discussions. It allows therapists to see firsthand the thought patterns and emotional responses their clients are experiencing, facilitating more targeted interventions. Moreover, seeing documented progress can be incredibly motivating for clients, reinforcing the positive changes they are making.

Trauma recovery is another area where thought records and journaling can profoundly impact. If you're processing traumatic experiences, these practices offer a safe and structured way to explore your thoughts and feelings. Guided by a therapist, journaling can help you work through trauma at your own pace, gradually building resilience and healing.

### *Thought Journaling Exercise*

Sometimes, all you need to do is journal your thoughts without following specific prompts. The following exercise can make you comfortable with thought journaling so you can do it daily:

Begin by finding a quiet space where you can sit comfortably. Take a few deep breaths to center yourself. Let your mind settle. This helps track your thoughts over time. Allow yourself to feel free as you begin jotting down whatever comes to mind.

Write about your day. Did anything interesting happen? Did something make you smile or upset you? Capture those feelings. Don't worry about grammar or punctuation. The goal is to let your thoughts flow. If you find your mind blank, write about the weather or how the music you're listening to makes you feel. This can help spark more ideas.

After you've written about your day, think about your goals. What do you want to achieve? Write down any goals you have, big or small. You can read more books or start a new hobby. It's okay if you don't know what you want right now. Writing can help clarify your thoughts.

Next, explore any challenges you face. Is there anything that has been bothering you? Could you write it down? A situation at work or something personal is on your mind. Describe it in simple terms. This can help you understand your feelings better. Don't hold back; this space is for your thoughts only.

Shift your focus to something positive. List three things you are grateful for. They can be simple, like a warm cup of coffee in the morning or a friendly chat with a neighbor. Gratitude can improve your mood and outlook. Reflecting on these things will brighten your day.

## Exposure Therapy Guidelines

Exposure therapy is a powerful method within CBT that addresses anxiety and fear through controlled, gradual exposure to distressing situations. Instead of avoiding situations that make you anxious and overwhelmed when they arise, you can be in more control. Here are some benefits of exposure therapy that make it a valuable practice to pursue:

- **Reduces fear.** One of the core benefits of exposure therapy is its ability to reduce fear through repeated exposure to anxiety-provoking situations. Whether the fear is related to specific phobias, such as a fear of heights or public speaking or more generalized anxiety, confronting these fears in a safe environment can significantly decrease the associated anxiety over time. For instance, if you fear dogs, exposure therapy might begin with viewing pictures of dogs, progressing gradually to watching videos, observing a dog from a distance, and eventually, interacting with a dog directly under controlled conditions. This slow but steady exposure helps desensitize you to the feared object or situation incrementally, reducing your fear response.

- **Builds confidence.** Addressing your fears and anxieties indirectly and gradually increasing your exposure to them can be a significant confidence boost for you. Starting with less intimidating tasks is crucial for building confidence and encouraging progress. In the initial stages of exposure therapy, it is essential to focus on manageable steps, because this can be counterproductive to confidence building. For example, someone with social anxiety might initially practice small, low-risk interactions, such as asking a stranger for directions or talking with a cashier. These smaller tasks help you build confidence and develop coping mechanisms before moving on to more challenging exposures. By achieving success with these less-daunting tasks, you can also gain the motivation and self-assurance to tackle more significant fears.

- **Minimizes anxiety.** Exposure therapy makes you a lot less anxious about your daunting fears as you realize your fears are manageable. Engaging in exposure therapy with a trusted support system can significantly minimize anxiety spikes during the process. The presence of a supportive friend, family member, or therapist provides emotional safety and reassurance, making you a bit more comfortable in an unfamiliar situation. This support system can offer encouragement, helping you stay grounded. They can also provide immediate assistance if your anxiety becomes too intense. For example, if you practice exposure therapy for your fear of flying, you might benefit from having a trusted companion during practice flights or simulation exercises. This person's presence can be a calming influence, making the exposure process feel less overwhelming.

- **Encourages longevity.** Documenting outcomes throughout the exposure therapy process can boost your motivation to continue. Keeping a detailed record of each exposure session, including your feelings before, during, and after the exposure, allows for reflection on progress over time. Journaling these experiences tracks your improvements and provides valuable information about yourself that helps you learn how your anxiety impacts you. For instance, a journal entry might note how initially looking at pictures of spiders caused severe anxiety, but after several sessions, the same activity only caused mild discomfort. Documenting this progress reinforces the effectiveness of the therapy, which provides you with a sense of accomplishment, encouraging you to stay committed to this journey despite the obstacles you may face.

Now that you know how beneficial this practice can be, here are some tips you can follow to maximize the benefits you receive from exposure therapy:

1. **Customize your approach.** It is beneficial to customize your approach to exposure therapy based on your specific fears and preferences. Using therapeutic strategies to address your triggers and comfort levels enhances its relevance and effectiveness. Furthermore, it acknowledges the unique nature of your anxiety, making the therapy more impactful. For example, while some people may respond well to imaginal exposure (vividly imagining the feared scenario) others might find in vivo exposure (directly

confronting the fear in real life) more beneficial.

2. **Implement helpful behaviors.** Implementing effective behavioral strategies can ensure the success of your exposure therapy. Therapists often employ techniques such as relaxation exercises, cognitive restructuring, and mindfulness practices to complement exposure activities. You can incorporate these same behaviors and activities into your daily routine. Relaxation exercises, such as deep breathing and progressive muscle relaxation, can help manage the physiological symptoms of anxiety during exposure. Cognitive restructuring involves challenging and reframing irrational thoughts about the feared situation, replacing them with more realistic and balanced perspectives. Mindfulness practices encourage staying present and focused, reducing the tendency to ruminate on anxiety-provoking thoughts. Incorporating these strategies can help you manage your anxiety both during and outside of exposure sessions.

3. **Keep your approach gradual and slow.** Gradual exposure to anxiety- provoking situations is the optimal approach when striving for change without overstimulating yourself. Jumping straight into highly distressing scenarios can lead to stress and potential setbacks. Instead, a systematic approach that progressively increases the difficulty level ensures you build tolerance at a manageable and realistic pace. This method, known as "graded exposure," carefully structures the exposure hierarchy, starting from less anxiety-inducing tasks and gradually moving toward more challenging ones. Each step serves as a building block, preparing you for the next level of exposure without causing undue stress.

4. **Use your support system.** When practicing exposure therapy, you may find that your anxiety spikes significantly because you're

facing things that you're fearful of. Friends, family, or therapists who understand your fears and goals can be an essential pillar of strength when you're overwhelmed by anxiety. Their presence can provide security and grounding, particularly during more challenging exposure sessions. For example, if you're undergoing exposure therapy for agoraphobia, you might start by taking short walks around your neighborhood with a trusted companion before attempting solo excursions. This support structure eases immediate anxiety and creates a sense of shared achievement and accountability.

As you follow these tips and create rules and guidelines that make you comfortable when practicing exposure therapy, remember to document all your experiences, including the good and bad moments. Noting your progress can help you stay committed to this process.

## Journaling Your Exposure Therapy

Exposure therapy can be even more effective and valuable when you use your journal to track and progress the emotions and thoughts you experience during this process. An effective way to journal your exposure therapy goes as follows:

It is essential to note your initial feelings before facing fear. Write down your fear, anxiety, excitement, or even hope. Capture the intensity of these feelings on a scale from one to ten. This helps you identify changes over time. When you face fear, refer to these notes to remind yourself of your starting point.

Next, describe the situation in detail. Where are you? What do you see, hear, and feel? Writing this down can help ground you and bring clarity to the experience. Use simple sentences to outline the environment and be specific about your reactions. Write what you think might happen as you prepare to face your fear. Are you afraid of judgment? Rejection?

|   |
|---|
|   |

After the exposure, reflect on the experience. Did it go as expected? How did your feelings change during the process? Note the moments when you felt most scared and how you handled those feelings. Include any positive outcomes, even if they are small.

Acknowledge the courage to face your fear and reflect on any steps you took that surprised you.

|   |
|---|
|   |

Set up goals for future exposures. What do you want to achieve next time? Break down larger goals into smaller, manageable steps. Write this plan in your journal to refer to it as you progress. Consider adding a timeline to remain accountable. Acknowledging more minor victories along the way is crucial for building confidence.

|   |
|---|
|   |

Ask yourself what you learned from the experience. Did you discover anything new about your fear? It wasn't as scary as you thought. Reflecting on these insights deepens your understanding and can motivate you for future challenges.

Write about your thoughts in a way that is easy to revisit later.

In addition to your reflections, consider including affirmations or phrases that encourage you. Write down things you want to remind yourself of during challenging moments, such as "I am brave" or "I can do this." These positive statements can serve as powerful reminders during future exposures. Reading them out loud can also help reinforce confidence and reduce anxiety.

You might also explore how your exposure therapy aligns with your broader life goals. How does facing this fear contribute to your personal growth? Reflecting on this broader connection can provide a greater sense of purpose. Write about your aspirations and explain how overcoming concerns can lead to reaching those goals. Another useful prompt is to discuss what support you need from your friends or family.

Are there people in your life who can help you? Write about how you'll ask for that support. This can include talking about what you are facing or how they can assist you. Emotional support from those close to you can make a significant difference.

Consider writing about distractions that could help you during moments of anxiety. What activities or thoughts can you turn to when you feel overwhelmed? List things that bring you joy or calmness. For example, you might listen to music, walk, or meditate. Documenting these strategies will provide you with tools to manage anxiety more effectively.

Use your journal to reflect on your overall mood after each exposure. Keeping track of how you feel over time helps you paint a bigger picture of your journey. Note changes over weeks or months.

Are you feeling more positive overall? Charting this progress shows that change is possible and motivates you to continue.

Throughout this process, remind yourself that it's normal to have ups and downs. Not every exposure will go perfectly, and that's okay. Write about the moments when things do not go as planned. Use these moments as learning opportunities. Reflect on handling disappointments and how they can lead to future growth.

# CBT for Anxiety Management

Anxiety is a common mental health issue that many people face, and CBT has proven to be a practical approach for managing anxiety symptoms. The following techniques of CBT showcase its ability to manage your anxiety:

- **Know your common triggers.** Triggers for anxiety can vary widely due to personal experiences, fears, and trauma. Common triggers include social situations, work stress, or even specific thoughts that lead to feelings of unease. Self-awareness is the first crucial step in managing these triggers. By identifying what sets explicitly off your anxiety, you can take proactive steps toward management. Keeping a journal to note down when anxiety hits and what is happening at that moment can be beneficial. Over time, patterns may emerge that provide insight into what causes the most distress. This self-awareness allows you to anticipate stressful situations and prepare coping mechanisms in advance.

- **Reframe your negative thoughts.** The most popular technique that makes CBT effective is reframing negative thoughts. If you experience anxiety or depression, you may tend to catastrophize or view situations in a very negative light. Reframing these thoughts involves recognizing irrational or overly negative thoughts and replacing them with more balanced, rational thoughts. For example, if you think, "I failed this task because I'm completely useless." Reframing could turn this into, "This task didn't go as planned, but it doesn't mean I'm incapable. I have succeeded many times before" (Pietrangelo, 2019). This thought process alleviates immediate feelings of failure and builds a more constructive mindset.

- **Share your experiences.** Sharing experiences can be incredibly therapeutic and empowering. Talking about your struggles with anxiety in a safe environment can foster empathy and understanding from others who may have similar experiences.

- Support groups, whether in person or online, can provide a network of individuals who understand what it's like to live with anxiety. This communal support can foster mutual encouragement and shared coping strategies. Sharing personal stories can also make anxiety less isolated, showing you and others that you are not alone in your experiences.

- **Work with a therapist.** There are multiple ways that you can work with a therapist to manage your anxiety. Guided discovery is another CBT strategy that can be used to manage stress. It involves working with a therapist who questions your beliefs and assumptions. For instance, if you constantly think you will fail at social interactions, a therapist might ask you to consider evidence contradicting this belief. Have there been instances where social interactions went well? What factors contributed to those positive experiences? Through this process, you learn to see your fears from different perspectives, which can be more helpful and less anxiety-inducing (Pietrangelo, 2019).

- **Explore ways to relax.** If you have anxiety, you may notice that you're always tense and find it impossible to calm down. Relaxation techniques, such as progressive muscle relaxation and mindful breathing, are practical tools for lowering immediate anxiety levels. Progressive muscle relaxation involves tensing and then relaxing different muscle groups. This practice can reduce physical tension and promote a sense of calm. Mindful breathing focuses on taking slow, deliberate breaths and paying attention to the sensation of breathing.

Both techniques can be integrated into daily routines and used during high-stress moments to maintain composure and clarity (McCallie et al., 2006). You can find detailed descriptions of these exercises, among others, throughout this book.

## *Role-Playing Exercise*

You don't have to stick to traditional anxiety-relieving exercises like the ones mentioned above. You can also get creative. Role-playing can be used as a CBT tool to manage your anxiety. It involves acting out scenarios that cause stress in a safe and controlled environment. This can be done with a therapist or a trusted friend. By rehearsing potentially stressful situations, you can explore different ways to respond and develop skills to handle real-life encounters more effectively.

This technique can reduce the fear of the scenario as you become more familiar and comfortable with it (Pietrangelo, 2019). Here are some role-playing prompts to follow or inspire your own:

- **Job interview scenario.** One person plays the interviewer, and the other is the candidate. The interviewer can ask questions like, "What are your strengths and weaknesses?" or "Why do you want to work here?" The candidate practices their responses while focusing on speaking clearly and confidently. After a few rounds, you can switch roles, allowing you both to experience the pressure of the interview spot. This helps normalize the stress of interviews and boosts confidence for future ones.

- **A conversation with a difficult person.** One person plays themselves, while the other acts as the disruptive neighbor, perhaps one who plays loud music at night. You can express your concerns using "I" statements, such as "I feel frustrated when the music keeps me awake." This exercise teaches how to address conflicts calmly and clearly, reducing anxiety in real-life situations.

- **Friendship breakup.** In this exercise, one person plays the role of a friend who wants to end their friendship with the other. This exercise encourages discussing feelings and setting boundaries, essential for maintaining healthy relationships. You can voice your emotions and negotiate terms such as staying acquaintances or deciding to part ways without resentment.

- **Networking at a social event.** One person acts as the host of the gathering, while the others approach to introduce themselves. You can practice small talk, asking open-ended questions, and maintaining a conversation. Such exercises help reduce the anxiety related to meeting new people and develop better social skills.

- **Speaking to a loved one about a medical issue.** One person plays the loved one, sharing their concerns, while the other practices delivering potentially distressing news, like having to undergo surgery. This activity helps you communicate complex topics and prepare emotionally for conversations that may happen in real life.

- **Practicing assertiveness in a group setting.** One person advocates for a suggestion at a team meeting, while others voice potential objections. You can rehearse, presenting your ideas clearly and responding to critiques without becoming defensive. The exercise allows you to build confidence in expressing your opinions among peers.

- **Receiving constructive criticism.** One person takes on the role of a manager providing feedback on a project, while the other practices responding positively and asking for clarification. This exercise can prepare you for professional situations where you must accept feedback gracefully and make improvements without taking it personally.

Feel free to experiment with different scenarios and adapt them to suit individual needs. The beauty of role-playing is in its flexibility. Role-playing isn't just for resolving conflicts or facing fears; it can involve light-hearted activities, such as pretending to be characters from movies or books. Engaging in these playful acts allows you to relieve stress and experience the lighter side of life while gaining confidence in your social skills.

Encouragement and positive reinforcement during these sessions can make them even more valuable. You can celebrate your wins when navigating challenging scenarios to reinforce the learning experience. Friendships are essential during these times, especially when struggling with stress and friendship or relationship conflict.

## *Personalized CBT Action Plans*

Creating personalized action plans by integrating CBT strategies can significantly enhance your results, because you can adjust your strategy to your specific needs. By practicing various techniques and recording their impact on you, you can identify what plan can give you optimal outcomes.

## *Personalized Plans Encourage Accountability and Targeted Action*

Personalized plans are crucial because they encourage you to take ownership of your journey toward emotional well-being. You approach this strategy with a more hands-on mindset as you put thought and effort into deciding what plan is best for you.

Doing this can make your unique experiences with CBT more meaningful and engaging. This sense of ownership promotes accountability, making you more likely to stick with the plan. For instance, if you struggle with anxiety triggered by social interactions, your personalized plan might include targeted strategies such as gradual exposure to social settings or practicing assertiveness in conversations. Focusing on individualized solutions ensures that plans and actions are made to address your specific obstacles directly when socializing.

Personalized plans also facilitate targeted action. Instead of a one-size-fits-all approach, these plans allow you to tackle issues that may not be involved in a regular CBT strategy. If negative self-talk is a significant problem, your plan might incorporate cognitive restructuring techniques that challenge and reframe these unhelpful thoughts. Targeting specific areas of concern makes your action plan more efficient and effective in fostering emotional regulation.

## SMART Goals Lend Structure and Purpose

Your SMART goals come into play when you start planning your approach to emotional regulation. Setting SMART goals helps you create a plan with a good structure and purpose that gives you a clear and attainable direction.

One of your bigger goals is to manage your stress through relaxation techniques. A SMART goal might be: "Practice breathing exercises for 10 minutes every morning for the next month to reduce stress levels." This goal is *specific* (deep breathing exercises), *measurable* (10 minutes daily), *achievable* (a manageable time commitment), *relevant* (addresses stress management), and *time-bound* (one month). These well-defined goals provide a clear roadmap, making tracking progress and staying motivated easier.

When you approach goals with a structure, you're more likely to follow through with them instead of treating them like empty goals or promises. Finding ways to set goals that suit you can help you stay accountable. Including them in your journal can also be an excellent way to keep track of the goals you set so that you can follow through with them.

## Regular Check-Ins for Reevaluation and Celebration

Another way to ensure that you stick to your action plan is to maintain momentum through regular check-ins. These check-ins offer opportunities to reevaluate your progress while celebrating the wins you've achieved. Doing this will keep you motivated and allow you to stay consistent.

During these check-ins, you can reflect on what works well and identify areas needing adjustments. For example, if your selected relaxation technique isn't as effective as hoped, reevaluate it and explore alternative methods such as guided imagery or progressive muscle relaxation. Regularly reassessing your plan ensures it remains relevant and practical, allowing you to adapt to your evolving needs.

Celebrating your successes, no matter how small, is equally important. Recognizing your achievements creates a sense of accomplishment and reinforces positive behaviors, because you want to continue the excellent work for more praise and celebration. For instance, if you successfully attend a social event without significant anxiety, acknowledging this milestone can boost your confidence and encourage continued engagement with your action plan.

## Supplementing Personal Efforts with External Resources

While personalized action plans are effective, additional external resources can provide more effective results. Seeking out workshops, professionals, or support groups offer extra support and tools that may be beneficial.

Workshops offer structured learning environments where you can deepen your understanding of CBT strategies and practice new skills in a supportive setting. For instance, a workshop focused on mindfulness could introduce participants to various meditation techniques, providing practical experience and expert guidance. Of course, professional advice should be emphasized more. Getting help from therapists, psychologists, or specific professionals can help you persevere through life's intense ups and downs.

Support groups offer the added benefit of community and shared experiences. Connecting with others facing similar challenges can give you a sense of belonging and much-needed emotional support. It's often encouraging to hear how people who are in the same position as you have navigated setbacks and celebrated wins because they offer valuable insights that can be applied to your journey.

Integrating these external resources into your personalized action plan gives you a holistic approach that promotes good emotional health. For example, regular participation in a support group might be a recurring goal within your plan, while utilizing an app for daily mindfulness exercises can keep you engaged and accountable.

## Journaling Prompts

After reading about CBT and the benefits that you can achieve from this practice, follow these prompts to end this chapter on a reflective note. These prompts can help you realize the power you have over your negative thoughts:

What specific thoughts have caused you distress recently? Write them down and examine each one. Do they reflect the reality of your situation? Challenge these thoughts by asking if they are based on facts or assumptions. How do these thoughts make you feel? Note the emotions that arise and consider how they affect your behavior.

Think about times you felt happy or calm. What thoughts did you have during those moments? Create a list of positive affirmations that resonate with you. These affirmations can serve as reminders of your strengths. Repeat them daily to build a more positive mindset.

Reflect on a situation that caused you anxiety. What were your thoughts in that moment? Write about how you reacted and wish you could have responded instead. Consider what steps you can take next time to handle similar situations better.

What are the common themes in your negative thoughts? Are there patterns that emerge when you examine them closely? Write down any recurring themes and consider how they affect your overall mood. Challenge the validity of these themes and brainstorm different perspectives to shift your thinking.

Identify moments when you felt proud of yourself. What thoughts or behaviors contributed to those feelings of pride?

Write about these moments and how you can replicate them daily. Use these experiences as motivation to counter negative self-talk.

## Summary and Reflections of CBT Techniques and Tools

In this chapter, we have explored the various tools that you can use to integrate CBT successfully into your daily life. From the engaging activities in behavioral activation to the informative reflections you discover through thought records and journaling, each tool offers actionable strategies to manage your emotions more effectively. Embracing these practices helps you experience a positive shift in your mood, reduce anxiety, and build a structured routine that promotes stability and predictability during challenging times.

As we wrap up this chapter, remember that the journey toward better emotional management is unique and personal. With consistent effort, you can improve your emotional and mental health.

Every action, whether scheduling enjoyable activities or documenting your thoughts in a journal, is a step toward greater emotional well-being.

Utilize these CBT tools as part of your daily life and, over time, you will likely notice improvements in how you handle emotionally challenging situations. Keep moving forward with patience and self- compassion, knowing that progress is still progress, no matter how small.

If CBT has provided some benefits but you'd like more actionable steps for emotional growth, dialectical behavior therapy is another excellent therapeutic approach. In the following chapter, we will explore what it is and set you up with the information that you need to practice it successfully.

# You're on a journey of self-discovery and growth, and we want to be there every step of the way. That's why we've included a special bonus:

This printable CBT and DBT skill tracker are designed to be your trusted companion, helping you stay focused and motivated as you learn and practice these powerful skills. It's like having a personal coach in your pocket, encouraging you to track your progress, set goals, and reflect on your emotional journey.

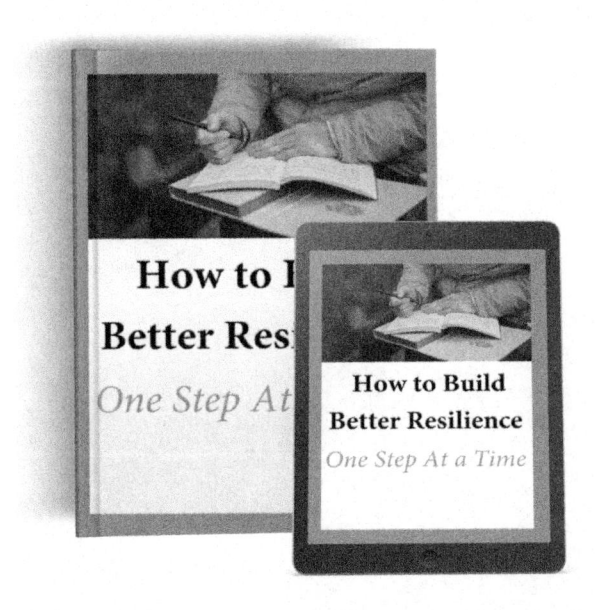

*Ready to take control of your well-being? Scan the QR Code to download your free copy now.*

# Chapter 3: Introduction to Dialectical Behavior Therapy

The next therapeutic strategy we'll unpack is dialectical behavior therapy (DBT). Understanding DBT begins with recognizing its unique blend of therapeutic techniques designed to address complex emotional and mental health challenges. DBT was initially created for those who have borderline personality disorder (BPD), but it is now popularly used as an effective mental health practice. After reading this chapter, you will have a solid understanding of DBT, including its origins, core principles, and ability to stand apart from other therapeutic models.

Within this chapter, you will uncover the theoretical underpinnings of DBT, tracing its development and the key concepts that drive its effectiveness. The fusion of mindfulness and cognitive behavioral techniques will be examined, highlighting how these elements work together to enhance emotional regulation, reduce harmful behaviors, and improve overall quality of life. We will also explore the dialectical nature of DBT—the balance between accepting yourself as you are and striving for meaningful change. Understanding these foundational aspects will give your insight into why DBT has become a vital tool in mental health, making it the perfect strategy for you and your mental and emotional well-being.

## Origins and Theoretical Foundations of DBT

DBT introduced a significant advancement in the field of mental health. Dr. Marsha Linehan developed it with the primary goal of treating individuals diagnosed with BPD. Linehan's journey in formulating DBT was deeply rooted in addressing the needs of highly suicidal patients, particularly those whose intense emotional pain often led to self-destructive behaviors. Historically, traditional behavioral therapies fell short of effectively managing these patients, making it necessary for a more specific and practical approach. This gap spurred the creation of DBT and its unique methodology.

One of the groundbreaking aspects of DBT is its integration of Eastern mindfulness practices with Western cognitive behavioral techniques. Mindfulness, a practice derived from Buddhist traditions, emphasizes living in the present moment with acceptance and nonjudgment. In DBT, mindfulness exercises help patients become more aware of their thoughts and emotions without immediately reacting. This practice lays a critical foundation for managing emotional responses, promoting a calm and centered state that facilitates better decision-making. All these aspects of DBT make it the therapeutic strategy it is today.

Interestingly, DBT builds upon the principles of cognitive behavioral therapy (CBT), but it enhances these concepts by integrating explicit training in mindfulness and emotion regulation. While CBT focuses primarily on identifying and altering negative thought patterns and behaviors, DBT emphasizes the importance of accepting your experiences, both good and bad, as a pathway to change. This dual focus addresses the immediate need for behavioral modification while fostering a compassionate understanding of the patient's emotional world. As a result, patients learn to challenge and change harmful behaviors and accept themselves and their circumstances, reducing the internal conflict that often drives maladaptive actions.

A core component of DBT is the debate between acceptance and change. This principle reflects the synthesis of opposing forces: The need for patients to accept themselves as they are while striving for personal growth and improvement. Acceptance involves recognizing and validating your feelings and experiences with understanding. On the one hand, when you feel accepted, you are more likely to engage in the therapeutic process and trust your therapeutic journey. On the other hand, the drive for change can motivate you to adopt new skills and strategies to cope with your challenges, which leads to meaningful and lasting improvements in your life.

## Four Modules of DBT Skills

DBT can help you approach your cognitive behavior while developing specific skills to effectively manage emotions, behaviors, and relationships. A crucial part of DBT is its focus on four fundamental skill modules: mindfulness, distress tolerance, emotional regulation, and interpersonal effectiveness. These modules structure this therapy, making it an excellent practice for mental health.

### *Mindfulness*

Mindfulness is a crucial component of CBT. It requires you to be fully present in the current moment, which is essential for understanding and managing your emotions. Mindfulness teaches you to observe your thoughts, feelings, and sensations without judgment. By doing so, you can gain a deeper awareness of your internal state, allowing you to respond to situations more thoughtfully instead of impulsively.

In practical terms, mindfulness can be divided into *what* and *how* skills. The skills include observing, describing, and attending activities with full attention. Observing involves simply noticing what is happening within and around yourself without trying to change it. Describing requires putting your observed thoughts into words, making the experience tangible and understandable. Participating means engaging fully in an activity and focusing entirely on the task.

The *how* skills encompass acting nonjudgmentally, one-mindfully, and effectively. Acting nonjudgmentally entails accepting things as they are without labeling them as good or bad, which helps reduce emotional distress. One-mindfulness means giving full attention to one thing at a time, enhancing focus, and reducing distraction. Acting effectively involves using skills and strategies that align with your values and goals.

## Distress Tolerance

Distress tolerance is another crucial factor of DBT, because it focuses on helping you survive crises without resorting to self-destructive behaviors. Life inevitably brings about pain and difficult situations, but distress tolerance prepares you with the tools and strategies to endure these moments healthily. The following critical strategies of distress tolerance can help you manage anything that life throws at you:

- **Radical acceptance** means acknowledging reality as it is without fighting it. It does not mean approving or settling for unfavorable circumstances but seeing things clearly and accepting their existence. This mindset reduces the unnecessary emotional strain caused by resistance to painful realities.

- **Self-soothing techniques** involve comforting yourself by practicing sensory experiences, such as taking a warm bath, listening to calming music, or engaging in a pleasant hobby. These activities help shift focus away from distress and promote calmness.

- **Crisis survival skills** are pivotal during extreme emotional turmoil. They offer immediate and practical ways to cope with overwhelming feelings. For example, the TIPP skills—temperature, intense exercise, paced breathing, and progressive muscle relaxation—can quickly alter your physiological state, especially if you're stressed. Another technique, *distracting with ACCEPTS*, involves using activities to allow your intense emotions to subside.

## *Emotional Regulation*

Emotional regulation is about understanding and managing intense emotions effectively. Learning the nature and functions of your emotions enables you to identify and label your feelings accurately. Recognizing triggers and the patterns of your emotional responses is a foundational step in emotional regulation. Understanding your emotions helps you manage them to reduce the stress that they potentially cause you.

A significant aspect of emotional regulation is learning to engage in behaviors contradicting harmful emotional impulses. For instance, if your anger prompts the urge to lash out, you can engage in a calming activity that counteracts your instinct to be aggressive. Regularly employing such techniques strengthens emotional resilience and allows you to develop much healthier long-term coping mechanisms.

Finally, increasing the number of positive experiences is vital for improved emotional regulation. Mastering this involves engaging in activities that enhance your skills and competence, boost your self-confidence, and reduce your vulnerability to negative emotions. Increasing the number of positive experiences consists of doing what you enjoy regularly.

## *Interpersonal Effectiveness*

Interpersonal effectiveness is the fourth module in DBT, which focuses on improving your communication and relationship-building skills. Successful interpersonal interactions require balancing three primary objectives: achieving goals, maintaining healthy relationships, and preserving self-respect. This balance ensures that you can assert your needs while respecting others' boundaries and keeping your integrity at the forefront of your decision-making skills. Effective communication strategies are central to this module. For example, DEAR MAN (Describe, Express, Assert, Reinforce, Mindfully, appear confident, Negotiate) provides a structured approach to expressing needs and desires clearly and assertively. This method helps you articulate your thoughts and feelings without aggression or passivity, promoting mutually respectful dialogue.

Maintaining relationships also involves using skills such as GIVE (Gentle, Interested, Validate, Easy manner). Being gentle and avoiding harsh criticisms, showing interest in the other person's perspective, validating their feelings and experiences, and interacting easily contribute to nurturing positive relationships. This practice inspires trust and collaboration, reducing conflicts and misunderstandings.

Balancing self-respect involves adhering to the FAST skills (be Fair, no Apologies, stick to values, and be Truthful). Treating yourself and others reasonably, apologizing less frequently to avoid undermining anyone's position, sticking to personal values, and being truthful even under challenging conversations bolster self-respect. Upholding these principles ensures that you meet your relationship and individual goals with your values and integrity prioritized.

## Self-Awareness and Mindfulness in DBT

Being self-aware and practicing mindfulness is an integral part of DBT. This self- awareness can encourage you to take control of your mental well-being by making better decisions. At its core, mindfulness involves staying present regardless of what's occurring around you and within your mind. This focus on the here and now significantly impacts emotional regulation.

Scientific studies emphasize the effectiveness of mindfulness practices in therapeutic settings. Research consistently shows that incorporating mindfulness into therapy helps decrease maladaptive coping strategies, such as substance abuse or self-harm. Intervention research has demonstrated that mindfulness-oriented therapies result in substantial improvements in psychological functioning, evidenced by reduced symptoms of depression and anxiety (Keng et al., 2011). These positive outcomes are attributed to mindfulness's ability to promote nonjudgmental awareness and acceptance of your experiences.

It's important to note that mindfulness practice is not limited to formal meditation sessions. It can be seamlessly integrated into daily activities, thereby enhancing its accessibility and practicality. Mindful eating, for instance, involves savoring each bite and paying close attention to the flavors and textures without distractions. Similarly, mindful walking encourages participants to feel the ground beneath their feet and notice the rhythm of their steps, promoting a grounded and tranquil state of mind.

The integration of mindfulness into everyday routines amplifies its benefits. When mindfulness is practiced consistently throughout the day, it becomes a natural part of life rather than an isolated activity. This ongoing practice strengthens the ability to remain present and attentive, which is particularly useful during stressful situations. By developing this mindfulness "muscle," you can handle emotional upheavals with composure and resilience.

Furthermore, mindfulness exercises extend beyond breathing and mindful movements, incorporating various techniques to foster self-awareness. Body scan meditations, where attention is systematically directed to different body parts, help recognize physical sensations and release tension.

Loving-kindness meditation, another valuable practice, involves sending goodwill and positive intentions toward yourself and others. This not only enhances emotional regulation but also cultivates empathy and compassion.

Applying mindfulness daily offers a practical guide for managing emotions effectively.

Consider the "STOP" technique:

- **S**top what you are doing

- **T**ake a breath

- **O**bserve your thoughts and feelings

- **P**roceed with intention

This simple yet potent method provides a structured way to cope with distressing emotions, allowing for a deliberate and measured response instead of impulsive reactions.

Adopting mindfulness in daily routines aligns well with DBT's goals of promoting a balanced life. You can create peace and clarity amidst a busy schedule by embedding mindfulness into ordinary activities such as washing dishes or commuting. This constant reinforcement of mindful practices ensures that the skills learned in therapy become ingrained, leading to lasting behavioral changes.

The symbiotic relationship between mindfulness and psychological well-being is supported by substantial evidence. Studies show that individuals practicing mindfulness report higher levels of self-reported mindfulness and improved clinical outcomes in conditions such as BPD (Eeles & Walker, 2022). By acting with awareness and healthy observation, mindfulness directly contributes to better mental health.

## Distress Tolerance Strategies

We discussed distress tolerance in a previous section but let's explore each of its techniques in more depth. The following methods can help you endure and cope with the stress and pain that often overwhelm you.

Although it's important to realize that your feelings are valid, you don't have to.

- **Practice crisis survival skills.** As you know, crisis survival skills are one of the critical components of distress tolerance. These skills provide immediate and practical means to handle extreme emotional pain, allowing you to navigate your crises safely. Taking a step back to calm down will enable you to approach your issues with a more leveled head. Taking a step back means physically or mentally removing yourself from the situational triggers, providing a momentary relief to think clearly. Observing your surroundings and internal state helps you understand your emotions and identify what triggered them. Proceeding mindfully involves acting to align with your long-term goals rather than short-term impulses (Survive a Crisis Situation with DBT Distress Tolerance Skills, 2019).

- **Introduce positive distractions.** Distraction helps shift focus away from distressing emotions, reducing their immediate impact. The ACCEPTS acronym in DBT outlines several strategies for distraction: activities (engaging in enjoyable tasks), contributing (helping others), comparisons (thinking about those worse off), emotions (inducing opposite emotions), pushing away (temporarily putting the situation out of mind), thoughts (shifting to other thoughts), and sensation (using sensory experiences). These activities can momentarily divert attention from emotional pain, creating a mental space to process feelings more calmly later (Sunrisertc, 2017b).

- **Endure stressful situations.** The IMPROVE technique in DBT offers another structured way to endure distressful situations. IMPROVE stands for imagery, meaning, prayer, relaxation, one thing in the moment, vacation, and encouragement. Imagery involves visualizing a peaceful place or imagining a successful outcome of the problem. Finding meaning in painful events often leads to personal growth and resilience. Prayer, or seeking solace spiritually, provides strength to face adversity. Relaxation techniques such as deep breathing or yoga help calm the body's stress response. Focusing on one thing at the moment prevents overwhelming thoughts about the past or future. A mental vacation imagining a serene place can provide a brief respite. Finally, encouragement through positive self-talk boosts confidence and perseverance (Sunrisertc, 2017b).

- **Avoid overuse.** Not all situations call for crisis survival skills. These skills should be explicitly used when facing immediate, intense pain or acting on emotional impulses that could worsen the situation. It's equally important to use these skills sparingly for everyday problems, which might require other DBT strategies for emotional regulation. Learning to decide when to practice these skills ensures they remain practical tools for actual crises (Survive a Crisis Situation with DBT Distress Tolerance Skills, 2019).

- **Accept your reality.** Sometimes, changing your situation isn't possible, so accepting it becomes necessary. This does not imply passivity; it means acknowledging facts and working within those bounds. Reality acceptance skills involve recognizing that some aspects of life are beyond control and responding proactively. This mindset reduces the perceived need for drastic, often harmful actions when faced with uncontrollable events. For instance, someone who has lost a job may initially resist the reality of the loss, leading to increased distress. By practicing acceptance, they can redirect their energy toward adapting to new circumstances, such as updating their resume or exploring new career opportunities.

  Accepting reality thus serves as a foundation for resilient coping, providing a stable platform to assess options and take constructive steps.

Finding skills that you can practice in times of crisis prepares you for any event that may come your way.

## DBT's Approach to Emotional Regulation

Understanding and managing emotions more effectively can be a game-changer for you, especially if you struggle with emotional regulation. DBT offers methods and practical tools to help you navigate your emotional landscapes. The following DBT strategies showcase why it's such a promising approach for practicing emotional regulation:

- **Understand the nature of your emotions and their triggers.** Emotions are complex responses to internal and external stimuli. They can encompass many experiences, from joy and excitement to anger and sadness. Identifying what triggers these emotions is a foundational step in emotional regulation. Triggers can be external events, such as a stressful work situation, or internal processes, such as negative self-talk.

- **Recognize emotional responses.** This starts with acknowledging physical sensations and thoughts associated with them. For instance, anger might manifest as a tightened jaw or clenched fists, while anxiety might present as a racing heart or sweaty palms. By tuning in to these cues, you can map out patterns in your emotional responses.

- **Learn practical skills to approach emotions.** Once these patterns are established, the next step involves practical skills for altering those responses. DBT introduces several exercises to help individuals change their reactions to emotional triggers. One effective exercise is the *Opposite Action* technique. When faced with a strong emotion, you are encouraged to identify the action that aligns with it and then do the opposite. For example, if anger pushes you toward confrontation, you might walk away or engage in a calming activity instead. This practice helps disrupt automatic reaction cycles and fosters more deliberate, healthier responses.

- **Stay open to different skills.** Another valuable skill is the TIPP technique, which helps manage overwhelming emotions quickly. Cooling down by splashing cold water on the face, engaging in short bursts of intense physical activity, slowly tensing and relaxing different muscle groups, and practicing deep, paced breathing can regulate physiological arousal associated with intense emotions.

- **Know the value of skill-building.** Strengthening emotional resilience through skill-building is another critical aspect of DBT. Resilience allows you to bounce back from adversity and cope with stress more effectively. One way in which DBT promotes emotional regulation is by teaching self-soothing techniques that engage the five senses. Listening to calming music, smelling a favorite scent, watching a beautiful scene, tasting a comforting drink, or touching a soft fabric can all provide immediate comfort in difficult moments.

Long-term benefits of strengthening emotional resilience include better mental health, improved relationships, and greater well-being. As you become more adept at managing your emotions, you will most likely find yourself more capable of handling life's challenges with grace and clarity. Emotional resilience not only helps in personal growth but also inspires healthier, more fulfilling connections with others.

## Journaling Prompts

Journaling is the best approach to practicing DBT and regulating nuanced and complex emotions. The following journal prompts can help you process the emotions behind this practice:

What emotions did I feel today? Write about the situations that triggered these feelings and how I responded. What was my physical reaction? Did I notice any changes in my body?

How did my environment affect my mood? Identify the places or people that influenced my emotions today. Did I feel supported or overwhelmed by my surroundings?

What thoughts ran through my mind when I experienced strong emotions? Write down any negative or unhelpful thoughts and examine their truthfulness. What positive affirmations can I replace them with?

What skills from DBT did I use today? Reflect on any techniques I practiced, such as mindfulness or distress tolerance. Did these skills help me manage my emotions effectively?

What do I want to learn about my emotional responses? Make a list of questions about my feelings that I want to explore further. What patterns do I notice in my emotional experiences?

Describe a time when I successfully managed a complex emotion. What did I do, and how did it feel to overcome that challenge? What can I learn from that experience?

What is a specific emotion I find hard to express? Write about why it's challenging and what I can do to communicate this emotion better in the future.

What are some of my coping strategies? List effective methods I use to cope with stress and emotional pain. Which strategies are healthy, and which do I need to change?

When I think of my emotional triggers, what comes to mind? Identify at least three situations or topics that consistently evoke strong emotional reactions. How can I prepare for these triggers in the future?

How do I feel about my progress in DBT? Write about any changes I've noticed in my emotional regulation and how I view myself since starting this practice. What are my strengths, and what areas still need work?

What are my goals related to emotional regulation? Write down my short-term and long- term objectives. How can I measure my progress toward these goals?

## Bringing It All Together With DBT

As we have explored throughout this chapter, DBT stands out for its unique blend of mindfulness and cognitive behavioral techniques. We discussed how DBT was developed to address the needs of people who struggle with BPD and its effectiveness in treating various other mental health conditions. DBT is a compassionate approach to managing your emotions and behaviors constructively.

The core components of DBT, including mindfulness, emotion regulation, distress tolerance, and interpersonal effectiveness, make it a mentally rewarding practice. These skills empower you to navigate your emotional landscapes more effectively, building healthier relationships. Understanding these principles helps with emotional regulation and offers valuable tools for personal growth and self-improvement, making DBT a versatile and impactful therapeutic approach.

This chapter taught you the basics of DBT, which makes it a valuable therapeutic strategy. The next chapter will explore this practice in more detail and uncover some practical DBT techniques and strategies.

**Managing stress and overwhelming emotions can be tough, especially when you're in the moment.**

That's why we put together this downloadable toolkit—to give you practical, on-the-go strategies that really work. Inside, you'll find mindfulness exercises, grounding techniques, sensory awareness practices, and quick interventions to help you stay present and navigate difficult feelings with confidence

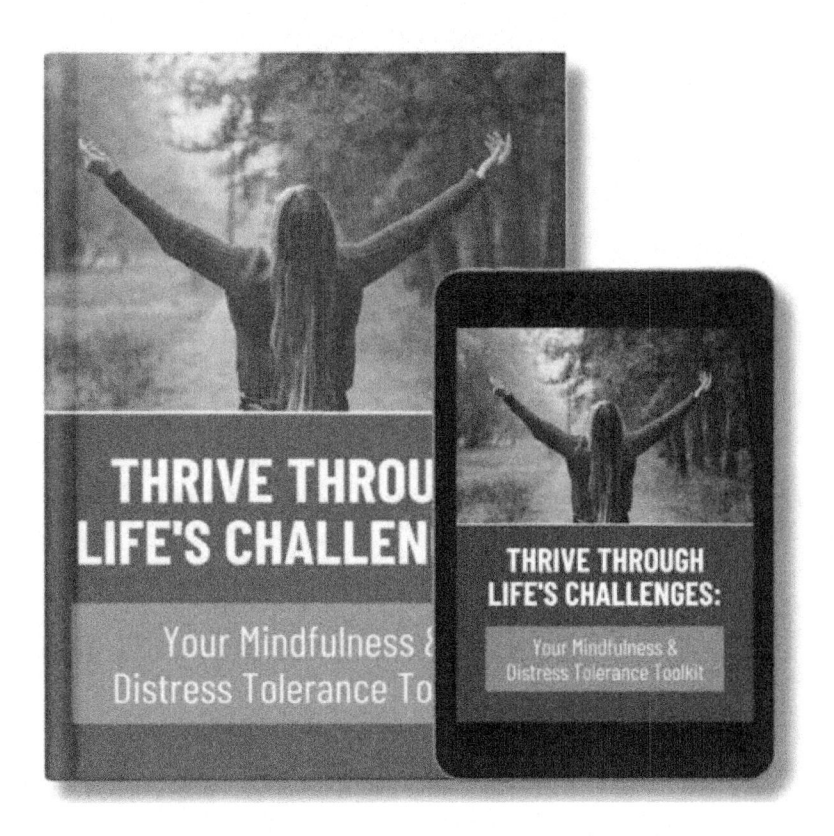

To download your free copy, simply scan the QR Code.
Take the first step toward feeling grounded today.

# Chapter 4: Practicing DBT Skills

Now that we know more about DBT, we must practice what we have learned. Practicing DBT skills requires a dedicated application of the techniques designed to improve emotional regulation and interpersonal effectiveness. You can better manage your emotions and foster healthier relationships by working through these skills.

This chapter contains practical daily exercises that you can implement, making complex therapeutic concepts accessible and actionable. These practices are not just theoretical; you're meant to engage in them actively. They offer a hands-on approach to personal growth and mental well-being.

In this chapter, we will discuss the various structured methods of DBT, which serve as critical tools for enhancing emotional and mental well-being. You will also learn how to assertively communicate your needs, reinforce positive outcomes, and handle rejection gracefully. This chapter also walks you through strategies for managing conflict constructively, ensuring that disagreements lead to understanding rather than discord. Practical tips and real-life examples illustrate how these techniques can seamlessly integrate into everyday interactions.

Using DBT diary cards introduces an alternative way of tracking emotional patterns and practicing self-reflection to reinforce the skills that you've learned.

Using the practical tips provided throughout this chapter, you will be able to enhance your relationship with yourself, which can, in turn, inspire you to nurture meaningful connections.

## Interpersonal Effectiveness Roles

Interpersonal effectiveness is an essential skill when practicing DBT. It helps you build and maintain meaningful relationships while communicating effectively. The following acronyms and exercises can help you tackle any conflict or issues in your relationships, allowing you to build stronger bonds that stand the test of time.

### Understanding DEAR MAN

One of the essential tools in DBT for interpersonal effectiveness is the DEAR MAN technique. As mentioned in the previous chapter, DEAR MAN stands for describe, express, assert, reinforce, mindful, appear confident, and negotiate. These components provide a structured method for asking for what you want or saying no to requests while respecting yourself and others.

- **Describe:** Start by describing the situation objectively without emotion or judgment. For instance, if you're asking for a raise at work, you might begin with, "I have been with the company for three years."

- **Express:** Clearly express your feelings and needs. Using the previous example, you could say, "I feel undervalued, given my contributions."

- **Assert:** Assert your request confidently but respectfully. An assertion could be,
"I believe a salary review is warranted based on my performance."

- **Reinforce:** Reinforce the positive outcomes of complying with your request. For example, you might add, "A salary review would motivate me to continue putting in my best effort."

- **Mindful:** Stay present and focused during the interaction, avoiding distractions. Repeat your request, if necessary, without getting sidetracked.

- **Appear confident:** Your tone, body language, and words should convey confidence. Even if you're nervous, maintain steady eye contact and a calm voice.

- **Negotiate:** If your initial request isn't acceptable, be open to finding a middle ground. Ask, "Can we discuss other forms of compensation or benefits?"

By practicing DEAR MAN, you can learn to ask for what you need and handle rejection gracefully, preserving your self-respect and relationships (Sunrisertc, 2017a).

## GIVE Skills

Maintaining healthy relationships requires more than being able to ask for what you want; it also involves effective communication that fosters empathy and validation. GIVE is an acronym in DBT for gentle, interested, validated, straightforward, and vital for sustaining positive interactions.

- **Gentle:** Approach conversations gentleness, avoiding harsh or abrasive language. This means being mindful of your tone and the emotions of the person you speak with. For example, instead of saying, "You never listen to me," try, "I feel unheard when my opinions aren't considered."

- **Interested:** Show genuine interest in the other person's perspective. Maintain eye contact, nod, and use verbal affirmations like "I see" or "Tell me more." Active listening demonstrates respect and attentiveness, making the other person feel valued.

- **Validate:** Acknowledge the other person's feelings and experiences. Validation might sound like, "I understand why you'd feel upset about this situation; it sounds tough." Validation fosters connection and reduces defensiveness.

- **Easy manner:** Conduct yourself in a relaxed and approachable manner. Use humor or a light-hearted tone when appropriate to ease tension. Smile and keep your body language open to create a welcoming atmosphere.

Both verbal and nonverbal cues play crucial roles in the GIVE skill. By embodying these principles, individuals can communicate more effectively and build stronger, more empathetic relationships.

## The FAST Approach

Balancing self-respect with the needs of others is another critical aspect of interpersonal effectiveness. The FAST approach in DBT stands for fairness, apology, sticking to values, and truthfulness.

- **Fair:** Treat others fairly and expect fairness in return. This means acknowledging the rights and needs of others while advocating for your own. If you're negotiating workload with a colleague, ensure that both parties' contributions and limits are respected.
- **Apology:** Apologize when you've done something wrong but avoid over- apologizing. A sincere apology involves acknowledging your mistake and expressing remorse without diminishing your worth. For instance, say, "I'm sorry for missing our meeting; I understand it caused inconvenience."

- **Stick to values:** Stay true to your core beliefs and values even when facing pressure. If you value transparency, don't agree to secrecy just to appease someone else. Upholding your values helps maintain self-respect and integrity.

- **Truthful:** Be honest in your interactions, avoiding exaggeration or deceit. Truthfulness builds trust and credibility. When conveying your thoughts, aim for clarity and honesty without being hurtful.

By employing the FAST approach, you can navigate interpersonal situations with integrity, ensuring that your needs and values are honored.

## Tips for Managing Conflict

Conflict is an inevitable part of any relationship. However, managing conflict constructively is essential for maintaining healthy relationships. Here are some strategies for resolving disagreements effectively:

- **Use "I" statements:** Frame your feelings and needs from your perspective to avoid sounding accusatory. Instead of saying, "You always forget my birthday," try, "I feel neglected when my birthday is forgotten."

- **Stay calm:** Keeping your composure is crucial during conflicts. Practice deep breathing or take a short break if needed to prevent escalation. Staying calm helps you think clearly and respond rationally.

- **Active listening:** Fully concentrate on what the other person is saying without interruption. Acknowledge what you hear to show understanding. For example, "It sounds like you're frustrated because you feel left out."

- **Seek compromise:** Aim for solutions that address the needs of both parties. Offer options and be willing to negotiate. For instance, suggest a new schedule that both find fair if arguing over chores.

- **Focus on solutions:** Shift the focus from blame to finding constructive solutions. Ask questions like, "How can we prevent this issue in the future?" Solution-focused dialogue promotes cooperation and understanding.

By implementing these techniques, individuals can manage conflict in ways that strengthen rather than damage their relationships.

## DBT Diary Cards

DBT diary cards are valuable tools to track your thoughts and behaviors. They are valuable if you aim to enhance your emotional regulation. Let's discuss how you can use diary cards to self-reflect regularly and commit to your DBT practice.

### Why Use Diary Cards?

Diary cards are a practical way to track and monitor your emotions, behaviors, and the usage of your DBT skills. These cards, which can be in paper or digital form, are a constant reminder to practice mindfulness and other DBT techniques, motivating you to be consistent with your self-improvement.

Diary cards are structured tools designed to help you track your day-to-day experiences. Each card typically has sections where you can rate your emotions, note any urges to use harmful behaviors, and check which DBT skills were employed throughout the day (Diary Cards | DBT Self Help, n.d.). Filling out a diary card encourages you to pause and reflect on your emotions and behaviors, inspiring a deeper understanding of your mental state and allowing you to identify patterns over time quickly.

This practice can contribute to significant improvements in managing anxiety, depression, or other emotional disturbances.

## *How to Use Diary Cards Successfully*

Using diary cards effectively involves several steps. Here are some factors to consider when using diary cards regularly:

- **Be consistent.** Documenting your experiences consistently is essential. Whether it's jotting down notes in the morning or summarizing your day before bed, regular entries ensure that you're keeping track of your progress accurately. It may feel tedious initially, but this habit becomes a part of your routine with time.

- **Be inspired by the benefits.** If you ever struggle to stay consistent, you may find it valuable to look at some key benefits that make this practice so powerful. These include increased self-awareness, better emotional regulation, and improved decision-making skills. Regularly recording your emotions and behaviors will teach you what triggers certain feelings and reactions. This awareness can inform better strategies to manage your emotions, leading to a more balanced and harmonious life.

- **Track your emotions.** Tracking emotions is a critical aspect of using diary cards. Emotions can be complex and multifaceted, so having a method to document them daily can provide clarity. Start by identifying your emotional experiences throughout the day. Were there moments of happiness, sadness, anger, or anxiety? If possible, write down these emotions and rate their intensity on a numerical scale. This quantitatively measures your emotional state over time, making it easier to recognize trends and triggers.

Remember that any progress is good progress. Be proud of yourself for the results you notice, regardless of how small they may seem. For example, if you see a decrease in the intensity of your negative emotions or a reduction in your harmful behaviors, acknowledge these achievements. Celebrating these small victories boosts your motivation to continue using DBT skills and maintaining your diary card entries. However, if you see recurring issues, use this insight to refine your strategies and seek additional support from your therapist or support group.

## Crisis Survival Techniques

When experiencing an emotional crisis, having the right tools and skills to manage overwhelming feelings is invaluable. DBT offers a range of techniques designed to help you tackle these intense moments and reduce impulsive behaviors. Crisis survival skills can be helpful in a variety of different circumstances. These skills are not about solving problems but getting through the moment without worsening things. Common triggers that can make use of crisis survival skills include relationship conflicts, significant losses, extreme stress at work or school, and other emotionally challenging scenarios. The following aspects and approaches of crisis survival can help you tackle any issue you come across:

- **Self-soothing elements.** These methods involve engaging the five senses— sight, hearing, smell, taste, and touch—to foster emotional stabilization. For example, during a crisis, a warm bath with a lavender-scented bath bomb can significantly soothe frayed nerves while listening to soft music. Eating a comforting snack such as chocolate or watching a favorite TV show can also provide immediate relief. The goal is to create a sensory experience that shifts focus away from distress to a calming environment, thus promoting emotional stability.

- **Distracting techniques.** As with defusion techniques, sometimes, the best thing you can do for yourself when you're overwhelmed and stressed is to distract yourself. Distraction is a practical approach within DBT.

These strategies help you redirect attention away from your painful emotions by engaging in alternative activities. Standard distracting methods include physical exercise, watching a movie, reading a book, or engaging in a hobby. The idea is to occupy the mind with something different and less emotionally taxing.

Activities such as doing a Sudoku puzzle or saying the alphabet backward can be particularly effective. They provide a mental challenge that diverts attention from emotional turmoil and helps avoid self-destructive behaviors until more rational thinking returns.

- **Radical acceptance**. Another indispensable skill set in DBT is radical acceptance, which teaches individuals to accept brutal realities without judgment. Accepting does not mean agreeing with or liking a situation; instead, it's about acknowledging reality as it is. For instance, if you lose a job, radical acceptance involves recognizing the loss without criticizing yourself or others for it. Personal stories and case studies often illustrate how accepting a harsh reality can lead to better emotional outcomes. A person might recount how accepting a chronic illness allowed them to adapt their lifestyle and find new joys despite their condition. Through these examples, you can learn that acceptance can pave the way for peace and resilience.

To showcase how these techniques genuinely work, it's valuable to consider real-life examples. Let's take Maxine's story, for instance. She found herself overwhelmed by anxiety after a significant life event. Using self-soothe techniques, she could gently calm herself by brewing herbal tea and lighting a scented candle. When her thoughts became too overpowering, she turned to distraction by walking briskly and focusing on the sights and sounds around her. Radical acceptance was pivotal in her journey, helping her cope with her circumstances without undue self-criticism. This holistic approach enabled Maxine to regain control over her emotions and navigate her crisis successfully.

These practical exercises underscore the value of learning and applying DBT skills in everyday life. You can effectively manage your emotional responses during crises by integrating crisis survival skills, self-soothe techniques, distracting methods, and radical acceptance exercises into your routine. The ultimate goal is to equip you with actionable strategies that promote emotional regulation and decrease impulsivity, fostering a calmer and more controlled approach to life's inevitable challenges.

To further enhance these teachings, providing structured guidelines for applying these skills is beneficial. For instance, when practicing self-soothing, you might start by creating a "comfort box" filled with items that appeal to your senses—such as scented candles, favorite snacks, soothing music playlists, and soft fabrics. For distraction techniques, you could list various activities you enjoy and keep this list handy for moments of distress.

## Validation and Self-Soothing Practices

Emotional validation and self-soothing strategies are joint when practicing DBT. Here's everything you need to know about engaging in self-validating and soothing techniques that make you feel better about the ups and downs of your emotional journey.

### The Concept of Validation

Validation is about recognizing and acknowledging your emotions without guilt or judgment. This practice is critical because it helps you feel understood and accepted, which can significantly reduce emotional distress. When your feelings are validated, you are more likely to experience relief and less emotional turmoil. Validation doesn't mean blindly agreeing with feelings; it acknowledges that those feelings are real and understandable given the situation.

Always be sure to validate your own emotions and accept validation from the people around you. To validate someone's emotions, start with active listening and empathy. Phrases such as "It makes sense that you feel this way" or "I understand why you might be upset" can be powerful tools for communicating validation. According to DBT principles, validation helps you regulate your emotions by decreasing the intensity of your negative feelings and developing a stronger sense of self-awareness.

### Practicing Self-Validation

Self-validation is just as important as validating others because it helps you accept yourself and the emotions you experience. It is about internally acknowledging your feelings and understanding that your emotions are valid and worth experiencing. This practice encourages a compassionate relationship with yourself, making navigating challenging emotional landscapes easier. Journaling some affirmations or Socratic questions and answering them can help you practice self-validation.

### Developing Self-Soothing Strategies

Self-soothing techniques are essential for regaining emotional stability. These strategies involve engaging in activities that provide comfort and relaxation, which helps reset your body's stress responses. Mindfulness exercises and grounding techniques are efficient self-soothing methods. Use the mindfulness activities we've discussed throughout this book.

Creating personalized self-soothing plans can make these techniques more effective. Identify activities that make you feel calm and centered, such as listening to music, walking in nature, or practicing gentle yoga.

Incorporating these activities into your daily routine can significantly reduce your stress.

## Skills for Balancing Acceptance and Change

While accepting yourself for who you are is crucial, you must balance this acceptance with actionable change. Life is about improving yourself and learning ways to cope during inevitably challenging times. Finding harmony between these two seemingly opposing forces is crucial to seeking healthy emotional regulation. The following is a comprehensive guide to integrating this balance into your life. Here are some important takeaways to consider when trying to balance these two elements:

- **Understand what debate is.** Understanding debate is the first step. In DBT, dialectic refers to the synthesis of opposites—specifically, balancing acceptance with the necessity for change. At the heart of this concept lies the *wise mind*. The wise mind is a state where you access both your reasonable (focused on logic and facts) and emotional (driven by feelings and impulses) mind to make balanced decisions. For instance, when faced with critical feedback at work, instead of reacting defensively (emotional mind) or dismissing it entirely (reasonable mind), the wise mind integrates emotions with facts to respond constructively.
- **Practice exercise.** Mindfulness exercises can be immensely beneficial in cultivating the wise mind. Utilize the mindfulness exercises described throughout this book, such as mindful breathing. The more you journal, practice mindfulness, and encourage self-awareness, the easier this therapeutic exercise will become for you.
- **Promote change.** Creating plans for change aligns with acceptance by focusing on personal growth while respecting your current state. Setting realistic goals is an integral part of these

plans. For instance, if your goal is to improve communication skills, you might set a SMART goal to join a weekly speaking club and track progress over six months. Tracking progress provides a sense of accomplishment and highlights areas needing adjustment. Using tools such as journals or apps can facilitate this tracking process, making it easier to monitor advances and setbacks alike.

- **Embrace your journey.** Embracing the journey emphasizes the importance of patience and self-compassion throughout the change process. Change is rarely linear; it often involves setbacks and plateaus. During these times, showing yourself grace rather than harsh judgment is essential. Understanding cultural narratives around change can also be enlightening.

- **Consider cultural influence.** Societal pressures often promote rapid, almost instantaneous transformations, setting unrealistic expectations. Recognizing this can influence a more patient and compassionate approach to personal development. Examining cultural narratives can sometimes reveal hidden biases about what constitutes "success" or "failure."

A more balanced view acknowledges that meaningful, lasting change often comes from sustained efforts and resilience. Learning from other cultures that value incremental progress and embrace lifelong learning can offer inspiring alternatives to your dominant narrative.

- **Be kind to yourself.** Lastly, grounding this journey in self-compassion is essential. Dr. Kristin Neff, a leading researcher in the field, defines self- compassion as treating yourself with the same kindness and understanding as a good friend. This is achieved by recognizing shared human experiences and responding to personal failures or difficulties with empathy. Self-compassion practices could include writing compassionate letters to yourself or engaging in self-soothing activities, such as reading a favorite book or taking a warm bath. Practicing self-care may be just what you need after having a rough day.

Consistent practice is the real key to achieving this balance of change and acceptance. The more you master this art, the easier it will be to integrate this healthy balance into your daily decisions and thought processes.

## *Journaling Prompts*

Here are some more journaling prompts you can answer for DBT practices:

What impact do my emotions have on my relationships? Analyze how my feelings affect the way I interact with others. Are there patterns I notice that I want to change?

What would I say to a friend who is struggling with similar emotions? Use this exercise to explore compassion and understanding. How can I apply this same level of kindness toward myself?

When I face a complex emotion, what are my first reactions? Describe how I initially respond to discomfort. Is that response helpful or harmful?

What have I learned about emotional vulnerability? Write about the importance of opening up and sharing feelings even when uncomfortable. What benefits have I observed from being vulnerable to others?

What are some of the myths I believe about emotions? List any misconceptions that I would like to challenge. What is the reality, and how can I shift my perspective?

What does it feel like to be in a state of emotional balance? Imagine what a calm and regulated state would look like for me. What can I do today to move toward that state?

What role does self-judgment play in my emotional experiences? Reflect on how harshly I critique my feelings. How can I practice self-compassion instead?

What recurring themes do I notice in my emotional journaling? Look back at previous entries. What patterns do I see that indicate my emotional growth?

How do I respond when I feel overwhelmed? Write about the techniques I use in those moments and whether they help me regain control.

What has been my biggest emotional challenge in the past week? Analyze what made it difficult and how I managed during that time. What lessons did I learn from that experience?

What is my relationship with anger? Explore how I express or suppress this emotion. Are there healthier ways to express outrage than I can practice?

How do I nurture my emotional health day by day? List small daily habits I can incorporate to support my emotional well-being.

What have I learned about the connection between emotions and physical health? Reflect on how stress or anxiety manifests in my body and what changes I can make to alleviate it.

What role does gratitude play in my emotional regulation? Write down three things I am grateful for and how focusing on gratitude can shift my mood.

What specific moments this week brought me joy? Record positive experiences and feelings that made a difference in my emotional state.

What boundaries must I set in my relationships to protect my emotional health?

Write about areas where I feel overwhelmed by others and what boundaries would help restore balance.

How do I feel about asking for help? Reflect on my comfort level about reaching out for support when needed. What fears or beliefs hold me back?

What emotions do I often try to avoid? Analyze why I hesitate to confront certain feelings and how to face them.

What techniques can I try to enhance my emotional awareness? List several mindfulness practices or exercises I can integrate into my routine to improve my emotional relationships.

What have my past experiences taught me about handling rejection? Reflect on how I react to perceived rejection and how I can better cope with those feelings.

How can I celebrate my emotional successes? Write about ways to acknowledge and reward myself for small victories in managing my emotions.

What do I hope to reflect on in my journal next month? Set intentions for the next few weeks regarding emotional exploration and DBT practice.

# Final Thoughts on Practicing DBT Skills

This chapter has uncovered various essential DBT techniques for enhancing emotional stability and healthier relationships. You can now better navigate your emotions and strengthen your relationships through the practical exercises and strategies discussed, such as DEAR MAN, GIVE, and the FAST approach, as well as conflict management tips. These skills provide an effective way for you to communicate, assert your needs, and maintain self-respect while being empathetic toward yourself and the people you interact with.

We also mentioned using diary cards as a valuable tool for tracking progress and self- reflection. Regularly documenting your emotions and behaviors and applying DBT skills can help you navigate the patterns and triggers that often influence strong emotional reactions. As you integrate these skills into daily life, you can expect to see meaningful improvements in managing your anxiety, depression, and overall emotional well-being. A practice that has similarities to DBT is acceptance and commitment therapy (ACT), which will be covered in depth in the following two chapters.

# Chapter 5: Introduction to Acceptance and Commitment Therapy

Acceptance and commitment therapy (ACT) offers a fresh perspective on managing emotional and psychological well-being. Unlike traditional therapies that often focus on eliminating distressing symptoms, ACT is all about embracing these thoughts and feelings, allowing you to understand yourself and the way you process your circumstances without feeling guilty.

In this chapter, we will journey through the critical concepts of ACT by providing practical tools and information that enhance your psychological flexibility, a crucial component for managing emotional well-being.

We will also explore the principles of this practice that make it so effective, including how staying present and adapting to life's challenges can reduce stress and anxiety. Learning how to practice ACT for emotional resilience will help you navigate challenging times with a calm and confident mind.

This chapter also highlights mindfulness practices, as with the other therapeutic strategies, because they provide essential techniques that influence awareness and reduce reactive behaviors.

Integrating these values into your daily life will drive your actions positively, allowing you to embrace your authentic self without letting negative thoughts overwhelm you.

## Principles of Psychological Flexibility

To understand more about ACT and its practice, it is valuable to examine psychological flexibility and what it stands for. Psychological flexibility enhances emotional resilience and promotes adaptive functioning. At its core, psychological flexibility involves staying present and adapting to challenges.

This adaptability allows you to reduce stress and anxiety by shifting your focus from unproductive worry about the past or future to constructive actions in the present moment.

Emotional resilience is strengthened when navigating life's adversities without becoming overwhelmed or stuck. When faced with stressful situations, having the capacity to adapt in the moment—whether by changing your perspective or behavior—can lead to lower levels of distress and a greater sense of control. For example, if you lose your job, you exhibit enhanced resilience and adaptability and can flexibly move forward by seeking new opportunities rather than dwelling on the loss.

However, factors such as past trauma and current stressors can impede psychological flexibility. These barriers can manifest as rigid thinking patterns, emotional avoidance, or automatic responses that no longer serve you. Past trauma might cause you to become hypervigilant about potential threats. At the same time, ongoing stressors such as chronic work pressure can drain emotional resources, leaving little room for adaptive thinking. Awareness of these barriers is crucial for developing effective coping strategies.

Recognizing these impediments can be the first step toward breaking free from maladaptive cycles and moving toward healthier patterns of thought and behavior. Some factors that can strengthen your psychological flexibility despite obstacles include the following:

- **Acceptance.** Acceptance is a big part of psychological flexibility. By accepting your thoughts and feelings without judgment, you allow yourself to experience the full range of emotions without being controlled by them. This nonjudgmental awareness creates space for personal growth and helps you develop a healthier relationship with yourself. For instance, acknowledging feelings of sadness or frustration without immediate attempts to suppress or change them can reduce your internal conflict and improve emotional regulation. Acceptance does not mean resignation but rather an acknowledgment of reality, which can empower you to take meaningful action aligned with your values.

- **Mindfulness.** Mindfulness practices also enhance your psychological flexibility. Mindfulness encourages being present and aware of your thoughts, feelings, and surroundings without immediate reaction or judgment. Techniques such as controlled breathing, body scanning, and mindful observation help you reconnect with the present moment and develop a greater awareness of your internal experiences. Regular mindfulness practice can diminish reactive behaviors and promote a calm response to stress. Mindfulness exercises can improve anxiety management and boost emotional resilience, even for a few minutes each day.

- **Values-driven behavior.** Engaging in values-driven behaviors can further enhance psychological flexibility. When you consistently act according to your values, you are more likely to make choices that align with your authentic self, regardless of external pressures or internal turmoil. For instance, someone who values family may prioritize spending quality time with loved ones despite a demanding work schedule. Acting in harmony with your values can provide direction and purpose, making it easier to navigate life's uncertainties. Over time, this alignment can contribute to a sustained sense of well-being and fulfillment.

- **Support system.** Building a support system is another practical step to enhance psychological flexibility. Social connections offer emotional and practical support, creating a safety net during difficult times. Seeking professional help from therapists or counselors is just as valuable because it can provide structured guidance and innovative coping mechanisms. A supportive network enhances resilience and encourages adaptive functioning by providing the encouragement and resources needed to overcome challenges.

## Understanding and Practicing Acceptance

Of course, acceptance is one of the main components of ACT. However, accepting yourself and your negative thoughts and emotions can be much easier said than done. Acceptance involves acknowledging and embracing thoughts and feelings without attempting to change or suppress them. Doing this makes you feel validated while providing practical ways to manage your distressing situations. Here are some principles of ACT that make it such a powerful practice:

- **Acknowledging that controlling your emotions often backfires.** One fundamental aspect of acceptance in ACT is recognizing that your attempts to prevent or avoid unpleasant thoughts and feelings often backfire. Avoidance strategies—distraction, suppression, or denial—might provide temporary relief but tend to exacerbate long-term suffering. When you avoid uncomfortable feelings, you inadvertently give them more power, allowing them to shape your behaviors and decisions in maladaptive ways. Conversely, accepting these emotions can lead to more adaptive behaviors. For example, someone anxious about public speaking might avoid it altogether, limiting their career growth. By acknowledging their anxiety, they can take incremental steps toward engaging in public speaking, thereby reducing the hold that anxiety has on their life.

- **Practicing mindfulness meditation** is an effective practice for cultivating acceptance. Originating from ancient traditions and popularized in modern psychology (Keng et al., 2011), mindfulness involves paying nonjudgmental attention to the present moment. Through regular practice, individuals learn to observe their thoughts and feelings without getting entangled in them. For instance, focus on your breath during mindfulness meditation and notice when your mind wanders. Instead of criticizing yourself for losing focus, you gently bring your attention back to your breath. Over time, this practice helps develop an accepting attitude toward your mental states, acknowledging them without trying to alter them.

- **Exploring structured exercises.** Structured exercises such as "noting" and "breathing into" discomfort are also methods to practice acceptance. Nothing involves mentally labeling your thoughts and feelings as they arise, like saying to yourself, "I am feeling anxious" or "I am thinking about work." This simple naming provides a sense of distance from your internal experiences, making them easier to accept. Similarly, breathing into discomfort involves directing your breath toward areas of tension or discomfort in your body, symbolically embracing the sensation rather than resisting it. These exercises can be integrated into daily routines, such as noting your emotional state during a stressful meeting or breathing into tension while commuting.

## *Naming Your Discomfort*

When you sense discomfort, both emotionally and physically, practice this exercise to name the feelings you're experiencing. Identifying them can make it easier to manage them.

1. When you feel tight in your chest, take a deep breath. Close your eyes if you can. Then, ask yourself what specific thoughts led to this feeling. You might think, "I feel anxious because I have a lot of tasks coming up." Write down that thought. Next, bring your attention to your body. Notice where the discomfort is strongest. Is it in your shoulders, your stomach, or your head? Name it. You could say, "I have a knot in my stomach." Acknowledge this sensation as authentic and valid.

2. Next, identify the emotions linked to your feelings. Maybe you feel overwhelmed, scared, or frustrated. Write these emotions down. Use simple words such as "sad," "angry," or "confused." This step helps create a list of feelings. Reading your list can make the emotions seem less powerful. You can say, "It's okay to feel overwhelmed." Normalize these feelings. Remind yourself that everyone experiences discomfort at some point. Now, think about when this feeling first started. Was it after a conversation, a specific event, or just a buildup of stress? Write down the moment. You could note, "I started feeling anxious after the meeting." This act of recollection helps you understand triggers. Understanding your triggers gives you a sense of control over the discomfort. You can think, "I can prepare for this next time."

3. Once you list your emotions and triggers, reflect on ways to address them. Ask yourself, "What do I need right now?" You may need a break, some water, or a chat with a friend. It's essential to identify what can ease your discomfort. Write down any ideas that come to mind. This gives you a plan. You may not say, "I should

take a walk," or "I need to talk to Alex." It transforms a sense of chaos into a structured approach.

4. Finally, each time you feel discomfort, repeat this exercise. Build a habit around it. Regular practice can make it easier to recognize and manage feelings over time. Share your feelings with someone you trust. Don't keep everything bottled up inside. You could express, "I'm feeling a bit overwhelmed," to a friend or family member. This sharing creates a support system, letting you know that you are not alone.

## Role of Mindfulness in ACT

As we've discussed, mindfulness is a fundamental aspect of ACT, which emphasizes being fully present in the moment and recognizing your thoughts and feelings without being hostile toward them. This practice helps you connect more deeply with your lived experiences, which inspires a more profound sense of awareness and acceptance. In ACT, mindfulness is about calming the mind and encouraging an open, curious, and nonjudgmental attitude toward internal experiences. Here are some techniques of mindfulness that can encourage effective ACT:

- **Breathing exercises.** One of the central techniques used in ACT to promote mindfulness is breathing exercises. These exercises encourage you to focus on your breath as an anchor to the present moment. Paying attention to the natural rhythm of breathing can cultivate a sense of calm and reduce the mental chatter that often accompanies stress and anxiety. Practicing mindful breathing regularly can enhance your ability to stay grounded and present during challenging times.

- **Mindful observation.** Mindful observation of thoughts is a crucial component of mindfulness in ACT. This technique involves observing thoughts as they arise without getting caught up in them or trying to change them. Instead of seeing thoughts as definitive truths, you can learn to view them as temporary mental events that come and go. This shift in perspective can reduce negative or distressing thoughts' power over your emotions and actions. Developing a more detached and compassionate stance toward your thoughts helps you effectively manage life's challenges.

- **Make intentional daily choices.** Being intentional about daily decisions is another critical strategy for incorporating mindfulness. This involves bringing a mindful attitude to routine activities such as eating, walking, or even brushing your teeth. By paying full attention to these activities, you can transform mundane moments into opportunities for mindfulness practice. For instance, while eating, you might focus on the food's taste, texture, and aroma, savoring each bite with full awareness. Doing this makes your everyday activities more enjoyable.

- **Use mindfulness to suit your needs.** Mindfulness exercises can also be adapted to fit your preferences and needs. Some might find structured practices such as meditation more appealing, while others might discover informal practices such as mindful listening or mindful speaking more appealing. Finding the right balance between formal and informal mindfulness practices can help sustain long-term engagement and make mindfulness a natural part of daily living.

The impact of mindfulness on mental health cannot be overstated. By fostering a nonreactive awareness of thoughts and feelings, mindfulness reduces the tendency to engage in automatic, habitual reactions that often contribute to stress and emotional distress. Instead, individuals learn to pause, observe their internal experiences, and choose more thoughtful and purposeful responses. This enhanced self-awareness and emotional regulation are critical components of psychological flexibility central to ACT.

## *Journaling Prompts That Inspire Mindfulness*

If you're having trouble with being mindful, the following journaling prompts can be answered daily to inspire mindful thinking and behaviors: What emotions am I feeling right now? Write down the feelings that come to mind. Are they positive, negative, or neutral? What triggered these feelings? Reflect on how they affect your day.

What is one thing I can appreciate about myself today? Write a positive trait or accomplishment, no matter how small. How does this acknowledgment make you feel? Each day, try to find something new to appreciate about yourself.

What am I grateful for at this moment? List three things, people, or experiences that you appreciate today. How do these elements influence your sense of happiness? Consider how gratitude can change your perspective.

How has my body felt today? Take a moment to note any physical sensations or discomfort. Are there areas of tension? Explore how these feelings connect to your emotional state. Acknowledge your body's messages.

What distractions did I encounter today? Write about moments when your mind wandered, or you were pulled into tasks. How did these distractions affect your ability to stay focused? Reflect on how you can gently redirect your attention.

How did I connect with others today? Write about interactions that felt meaningful or supportive. How did these connections enhance your sense of belonging? Consider the importance of fostering these relationships.

What did I learn today? Reflect on a new insight or understanding gained from experiences or conversations. How can this knowledge influence your daily life? Embrace opportunities for continual learning.

How did I handle challenges today? Think about a specific problematic situation you faced. How did you respond? What strategies can you use in the future to approach challenges mindfully and effectively?

What self-limiting beliefs did I notice today? Identify thoughts that held you back or made you doubt yourself. How can you replace these thoughts with more empowering ones? Challenge the stories you tell yourself.

What positioned me in a state of flow today? Write about moments when you felt fully engaged and present in an activity. How can you recreate this feeling in your daily life? Seek more activities that allow you to lose track of time.

What is my intention for tomorrow? Consider how you want to approach the day ahead. What mindset or attitude will guide your actions? Setting intentions can help shape your daily experiences.

Where did I find moments of stillness? Reflect on times during your day when you paused for a moment. What did you notice during these still moments? Embrace the power of pause in a hectic world.

What do I want to let go of? Identify any burdens, worries, or negative feelings that weigh you down. How can you actively release these from your mind and body? Letting go often opens space for new possibilities.

What was one moment today that felt perfect? Think about a time when everything seemed right, even for a second. What contributed to this feeling? Seek to recreate these perfect moments in your daily life.

How did I nurture my creativity today? Think about moments when you expressed yourself artistically or innovatively. What did you create or think about? Make space in your life for creativity to blossom.

How do I feel about social media today? Reflect on your experience with social media and its effects. Did it leave you feeling connected or drained? Consider setting boundaries to cultivate a healthier relationship with technology.

How can I be more mindful during meals? Think about your eating habits. Are you fully present when you eat? Consider practicing mindful eating by savoring each bite and noticing the flavors and textures.

How can I create a peaceful environment? Consider your surroundings and how they impact your mood. What changes can you make to foster a sense of calm? A quiet space can enhance your understanding of mindfulness.

How do I want to feel at the end of the day? Write down emotions you hope to experience by the day's end. What actions can you take to support these feelings? Setting a daily intention can help steer your experiences positively.

## **Values-Driven Life Planning**

Understanding and living according to your core values is a fundamental aspect of ACT. Values are guiding principles that shape our decisions and behaviors, leading to a more authentic life. Recognizing these values clarifies setting goals and ensures our steps align with what truly matters to us. Here are some ways you can live a more value-driven life:

- **What are values?** First, it's essential to understand what values are and why they matter. Values act as a compass, directing your actions and decisions toward what you consider important. They reflect your deepest beliefs and priorities and serve as a lens through which you view the world. When you live by your values, your actions feel meaningful, and you experience a sense of purpose. Conversely, you may feel disconnected or dissatisfied when your behaviors are misaligned with your values.

- **What are your values?** Several techniques can be beneficial in discovering your core values. Reflective journaling, for instance, allows you to explore your thoughts and emotions in depth. By regularly writing about experiences, reactions, and decisions, you can identify recurring themes that highlight what is important to you. According to Wright (2023, para. 23), "Reflective journaling offers a chance to identify what you value and believe clearly." This practice fosters self-awareness and helps clarify values over time.

- **How can you practice your values?** Another effective technique is the use of value cards. These cards typically contain shared values such as honesty, creativity, and compassion. You can sort through the cards, selecting the values that resonate most. This exercise helps identify and prioritize core values, offering a clearer understanding of what drives your actions. Using values clarification worksheets can provide structured guidance in this process by helping you select and rank your most important values (Selva, 2018).

- **How can you integrate values in groups?** Group discussions are also beneficial in uncovering core values. Conversations about values can reveal insights and perspectives that might not emerge in solitary reflection. Sharing experiences and hearing others articulate their values can help refine your understanding. Group settings provide a supportive environment where participants can collectively explore and affirm their values.

- **How can you live by your values?** Living in alignment with your core values has profound benefits. It increases motivation and resolve because actions aligned with values feel intrinsically rewarding. When you pursue goals that resonate with your values, you are more likely to stay committed and persevere, even in the face of challenges. Additionally, when your values align with those of others, it fosters a sense of community and connection. Being part of a group that upholds shared values can enhance feelings of belonging and support.

- **How does this boost your emotional well-being?** Understanding and living by your values can reduce internal conflict and provide a stable foundation during difficult times. It allows you to navigate life's challenges with a sense of direction and purpose. For instance, someone who values resilience might approach setbacks as opportunities for growth rather than obstacles. This perspective shift can significantly improve your coping with stress and adversity.

When you put your values first, you can always go right with decision-making. Although you may be influenced to make decisions that you don't necessarily enjoy, they will most likely be good for you and the path ahead of you (Wright, 2023).

## *Journaling Prompts*

You may struggle to find that balance between acceptance and commitment. The following journal prompts can help you practice ACT more effectively with self- compassion:

What does acceptance mean to you right now? Write down your thoughts and feelings about this concept. Consider times when you found it hard to accept something. How did you respond? What did you learn from that experience?

When you think about commitment, what comes to mind? Jot down your thoughts about commitment in your life. Are there areas where you feel fully committed? Are there places where you struggle? Explore the emotions tied to these feelings.

Reflect on a recent situation in which you felt overwhelmed. What thoughts ran through your mind at that moment? Write a detailed account of how you reacted. Did your reactions align with your values.
How might understanding your emotions impact your response next time?

Identify a value that's important to you. Write about why this value matters in your life. How does it guide your decisions? Are there moments when you have stayed true to this value, even when it was difficult?

Imagine a future where you are living in alignment with your values. What does that look like to you? Describe the actions you would take, how you would feel, and the relationships you would nurture. Let this vision inspire you and guide your journey.

Think about any fears that hold you back from commitment. What are they? Write them down. Challenge these fears by questioning their validity and how they affect your choices. Are your fears based on facts or assumptions?

Explore a time when you accepted a setback in your life. How did you handle the situation? What did acceptance teach you about resilience? What positive changes emerged from this experience?

Consider your self-talk when facing challenges. What kind of messages do you tell yourself? Are they supportive or critical? Write a dialogue between your critical voice and a kinder, more compassionate voice. How can you nurture the compassionate one?

Focus on a recent decision you made. What were the factors that influenced your choice? How did your values play a role? Reflect on whether you feel satisfied with the decision or wish to have acted differently.

List three things you are grateful for today. Reflect on how gratitude impacts your mental well-being. In what ways can you make gratitude a regular part of your life?

Describe a self-care practice that you find helpful. How does this practice support your mental health? Write about why it's essential and how you can prioritize it.

Think about your support system. Who are the people you can lean on? Write about the qualities that make them supportive. How do they help you navigate acceptance and commitment in your life?

Reflect on the concept of mindfulness. How can being more present improve your ability to accept complicated feelings? Write down a simple mindfulness technique and how it might help you.

# Final Thoughts on ACT as a Practice

In this chapter, we have explored the foundational principles of ACT and its unique focus on psychological flexibility. By understanding and practicing acceptance, you can face your emotions without judgment or avoidance, which is crucial for improving emotional resilience and overall well-being.

Mindfulness practices, such as controlled breathing and body scanning, significantly enhance your ability to stay present and manage stress. Engaging in values-driven behaviors helps you act in alignment with your core beliefs, contributing to a more fulfilling and authentic life.

Recognizing such barriers as past trauma and ongoing stressors is essential for developing effective coping strategies. Through awareness and acceptance, you can navigate life's adversities more effectively. Building a support system offers emotional and practical guidance, making it easier to overcome challenges.

ACT provides valuable tools for separating yourself from distressing thoughts, promoting greater emotional clarity and decision-making. Integrating these practices into your daily routines helps cultivate a mindset of openness and psychological flexibility, fostering long-term mental health and personal growth. After learning about ACT and what it stands for as a practice, it's time to engage in activities that can provide ample benefits and emotional growth. In the following chapter, we will cover ACT techniques.

# Chapter 6: Applying ACT Techniques

Applying ACT techniques involves learning to embrace your thoughts and emotions without judgment and make conscious choices aligned with your values. ACT empowers you to fully experience your mental and emotional thought processes while committing to actions that promote more meaningful behaviors.

This chapter offers practical exercises to implement these strategies effectively, helping you integrate ACT methodologies into your daily routine.

We'll also look into tangible exercises that make the principles of ACT accessible and actionable. You'll learn to enhance your awareness and presence in everyday activities through mindfulness practices such as breathing and body scan meditation. We will also focus on identifying and developing your values through guided reflections and vision board activities.

You'll discover exercises designed to encourage acceptance and willingness, which enables you to face uncomfortable emotions with resilience. Finally, additional cognitive defusion techniques will be covered to help you detach yourself from intrusive thoughts that may be taking a toll on your emotional regulation and overall happiness. This chapter will provide you with all the necessary exercises and support to thrive in any circumstance.

# Everyday Mindfulness Exercises

Throughout this book, we've discussed mindfulness practices rooted in most therapeutic practices. You can always integrate mindfulness practices into your daily routines because they can significantly enhance your awareness and emotional understanding. This section will explore practical ways to introduce mindfulness into your daily routine. The more often you practice it, the more mindfulness will become a natural part of your psyche.

## *Mindful Breathing*

Using your breath as an anchor is one of the simplest yet most powerful ways to stay present. Mindful breathing is about paying attention to your breath moving in and out of your body. Breathing deeply with intention helps you observe your thoughts without judgment, guilt, or negativity. It's an easy and accessible way to take control of your mind and body when you start to feel overwhelmed. Follow these steps to practice mindful breathing:

1. To begin, find a quiet place to sit or lie down comfortably.
2. Close your eyes if that feels right for you.
3. Focus on the sensation of your breath entering and leaving your nostrils.
4. If your mind wanders, gently bring your focus back to your breath.
5. Start practicing for 3–5 minutes, gradually increasing the time as you become more comfortable (Mayo Clinic Staff, 2020).

Consistency is critical for mindfulness to be effective. Mindful breathing is well worth the effort required. It helps calm your mind, reduce stress, and improve focus. If you're struggling with anxiety or depression, this practice can provide a moment of peace and clarity amidst the chaos of overwhelming thoughts and emotions.

Regularly practicing mindful breathing can lead to a heightened sense of control over your mental state, making it easier to get through those difficult times.

## Body Scan Meditation

Another effective mindfulness practice is body scan meditation. This popular exercise helps you tune into your bodily sensations, allowing you to develop a deep connection. Here are some steps you can follow to perform a body scan meditation:

1. Lie in a comfortable position with your legs extended, your arms at your sides, and your palms facing up.

2. Slowly bring your attention to each body part, starting from your toes and moving up to your head.

3. Notice any sensations, emotions, or thoughts associated with each part of your body.

4. Focus on each area for about 20–30 seconds before moving on to the following (Mayo Clinic Staff, 2020). This practice promotes relaxation and body awareness and alleviates physical tension. It's especially beneficial if you experience chronic pain or stress-related tension in your body. By regularly performing body scan meditation, you can develop a greater appreciation for your body's signals, leading to better self-care and a more balanced life.

## Mindful Eating

Eating, an activity you do multiple times a day, can be an opportunity for growth. Mindful eating involves fully engaging in the experience of eating, from savoring taste to appreciating texture to increase awareness of emotional triggers related to food. You may often eat while distracted by television, work, or other activities, leading to overeating and a lack of enjoyment. Here are some ways in which you can practice mindful eating to ensure that you enjoy your food more:

1. To practice mindful eating, start by choosing a meal or snack and sit in a calm environment free from distractions, including the television, your phone, or any other distractions that cause you to eat your food without intention.

2. Before taking a bite, pause and look at your food. Notice its colors, textures, and aromas.

3. As you eat, chew slowly and pay attention to the taste and texture of your food. Try to identify different flavors and sensations.

4. Notice how your body feels as you eat and identify hunger or fullness cues.

The benefits of mindful eating extend far beyond improving digestion and promoting healthy eating habits. Mindful eating can also help you recognize emotional triggers from unhealthy eating behaviors. By developing a conscious relationship with food, you can better manage your cravings and make more intentional dietary choices, creating a holistically healthier lifestyle.

## *Walking Meditation*

Walking is not only great for its physical health benefits, but it's also an opportunity to be more aware of your current reality and surroundings. Walking meditation offers an easily accessible way to integrate mindfulness into daily routines. This practice can be done by focusing on the rhythm of your steps and breathing as you work while letting nature enhance your awareness. Here are some steps to help you understand how to practice mindful walking:

1. First, find a quiet place to walk undisturbed for about 10–20 feet.

2. Stand still momentarily and take a few deep breaths, grounding yourself in the present.

3. Slowly start walking, paying attention to each step.

4. Notice the sensation of your feet touching the ground, the movement of your legs, and the rhythm of your breath.

5. When you reach the end of your path, turn around and continue walking, maintaining awareness of your sensations.

6. As you draw your attention to your body, consider shifting this focus to your beautiful surroundings, especially when walking in nature.

Walking meditation allows you to connect with your environment in a meaningful way. It can be particularly soothing in an outdoor setting you connect with. Listening to the birds chirping, feeling the breeze, and observing the play of light and shadow can deepen your mindfulness practice. This exercise enhances your awareness by giving you a gentle form of physical activity, contributing to your overall well-being.

You can cultivate a greater sense of presence and awareness by weaving these mindfulness practices into your daily routine. Start with short sessions and gradually increase the duration to make it easier for you to incorporate these exercises consistently. Whether you practice mindful breathing, body scan meditation, mindful eating, or walking meditation, each technique offers unique benefits that contribute to mental clarity and emotional resilience. Regular practice will help you integrate mindfulness into your everyday mindset.

# Identifying and Developing Your Values

Whether we're aware of them or not, we all have a set of underlying personal values that often influence our decisions. Understanding and committing to these core values are vital aspects of living an authentic and fulfilling life.

Core values act as a compass, guiding our decisions, shaping our actions, and providing a sense of direction and purpose. Learning about your values and creating a list that resonates with you will help you have a more successful experience with ACT.

## Values Exploration Exercise

The values exploration exercise encourages you to practice deep reflection to distinguish between societal expectations and personal desires. Here are some quick and easy steps that will help you identify your values:

1. To begin, find a quiet space to focus without interruption.

2. Reflect on moments in your life that significantly impacted you, whether positive or negative. These experiences often reveal what is most important to you.

3. Engage in self-reflection by answering the following questions:

    a. What activities or experiences make me feel alive and energized?

    b. Which qualities do I admire in others and which do I detest?

By exploring these questions, you can separate your desires from societal influences and uncover the core values that resonate most deeply with you.

## Values Hierarchy Creation

Once you have identified potential values, creating a hierarchy helps you prioritize them, providing a clear framework for decision-making. Start by listing all the values that emerged from the exploration exercise. Next, narrow down this list to the top ten values most important to you. Rank these values in order of importance, from most to least significant.

For example, if "family," "integrity," and "creativity" are among your top values, determine which one holds the most weight in guiding your decisions. Ask yourself which value you would prioritize if they ever came into conflict.

This process clarifies your priorities and helps ensure your life choices align with your most profound principles.

## Vision Board Activity

The vision board activity engages creative expression to visualize values and serves as a daily reminder of commitments. Gather magazines, photos, art supplies, and a board or large paper. Identify images and words that symbolize your core values and goals. Arrange these items on your vision board in a way that is visually appealing and meaningful to you.

For example, if "health" is a core value, you might include pictures of people exercising, fresh fruits and vegetables, or nature scenes that evoke wellness. If "career success" is essential, you might add images related to professional achievements or inspirational quotes about perseverance. Display your vision board in a place where you will see it daily. This constant reminder reinforces your commitment to living in alignment with your values, keeping them at the forefront of your mind.

## Check-In Process

A regular check-in process assesses alignment with personal values to strengthen authentic living. Schedule periodic check-ins, whether weekly, monthly, or quarterly, to evaluate how well your actions and choices reflect your core values. During these check- ins, ask yourself: Have my recent decisions and actions aligned with my values? Where have I fallen short, or in what areas have I faced challenges? What adjustments can I make to better align with my values?

For instance, if "balance" is a core value and you have been overwhelmed with work at the expense of personal time, consider changes that could restore balance to your life. This may mean setting boundaries around work hours or scheduling regular leisure activities. These check-ins serve as a compass, helping you navigate life's complexities while staying true to your core principles.

Living by your values can be challenging, especially in a world filled with competing demands and distractions. However, you can better understand what truly matters to you by undertaking these exercises—values exploration, hierarchy creation, vision board activity, and regular check-ins. This clarity empowers you to make decisions that lead to a more authentic and fulfilling life.

## Values Journaling Prompts

Along with the exercise and points that you read through in this section, follow some of these journal prompts further to identify your values and their significance to you.

What values do you hold dear? Think about the times when you felt joy or fulfillment. What was happening in those moments? Write about instances when you felt proud of yourself.

Who were you with, and what did you do? This could reveal values linked to relationships or accomplishments.

Reflect on your role models. Who do you admire, and why do you admire them? Consider what qualities they possess that resonate with you. Are they kind, driven, creative, or supportive? These traits might shine a light on your core values.

Think about the times you felt frustrated or upset. What triggered those feelings? Were there moments when your beliefs were challenged?

Identify what you stand for. Write about issues that matter to you, such as environmental conservation, education, or community service. Explore why these topics resonate with you. What experiences in your life have shaped these beliefs?

Consider how you spend your time and energy. What do you prioritize daily? Your choices reflect your values whether family, work, health, or hobbies. Are there activities that make you lose track of time? Describe those experiences. What about them that bring you joy. This can highlight what is the most important to you.

Think about what makes you feel fulfilled. Is it helping others, creating art, or solving problems? Write down your thoughts whenever you feel a strong emotional response. This can show you what you truly value. Reflect on your successes and failures. Write about what you learned from each.

Did your failures teach you resilience or perseverance? Did your successes make you more compassionate or grateful? These lessons often reveal deeper values.

Look back at your upbringing. What values were instilled in you growing up? Did your family emphasize honesty, hard work, or kindness?

Write about how these early lessons still influence you and how you live today. Are there family traditions that reflect these values? Jot down how they resonate with you now.

Imagine your ideal life. What does it look like? What values are at the center of that vision? Write about the person you wish to become. What qualities do you aspire to develop? This vision can help clarify what is most significant to you.

Focus on the impact you want to make in the world. How do you want to be remembered? Write about the legacy you hope to leave behind.

Consider your passions. What activities make you feel alive? Whether it's crafting, sports, or advocacy, your passions are often tied to your values. Explore how they influence your choices and relationships.

List moments when you felt truly connected to something. Identify what those moments had in common. Did they align with your beliefs or interests?

Think about the people in your life. Who are your closest friends, and what traits do they embody? Could you write down the values they represent? Are they loyal, optimistic, or adventurous? Reflect on how these relationships influence your values.

Consider the challenges you've faced. What values helped you overcome those obstacles? How did they guide your decisions during challenging times?

Think of the role community plays in your life. What does it mean to belong? Write about your involvement in community activities or groups. Do they reflect your values of service, cooperation, or learning? Identify how these experiences shape your worldview.

Set goals related to your values. What steps can you take to align your actions with your beliefs? Write down short-term and long-term objectives that resonate with you.

Explore the idea of balance. Are there areas of your life where you need to focus more on your values? Write about how you can create a more harmonious life.

Think about the words you use to describe yourself. Do they reflect your values? Write affirmations that resonate with your beliefs and aspirations.

Lastly, allow yourself to evolve. Recognize that values may shift over time as you grow and experience new things. Write about how your values have changed and what prompted those shifts.

Cherish your journey of self-discovery. Each prompt brings you closer to understanding and embracing your values.

## Acceptance and Willingness Exercises

Acceptance and willingness are the cornerstones of ACT. By embracing these principles, you can build resilience to face uncomfortable thoughts and emotions. The following points and quick exercises can help you accept yourself and inspire a willingness that motivates you to be the best version of yourself.

### Acceptance Journaling Exercise

One practical way to cultivate acceptance is through journaling. The acceptance journaling exercise encourages individuals to process unwanted emotions by providing structured writing prompts. Begin by selecting a quiet time each day to sit with your journal. Write freely about any uncomfortable feelings or thoughts you experienced that day. Reflect on how these emotions affected your behavior and interactions with others.

For example, if you felt anxious in a social situation, describe that anxiety in detail. What physical sensations did you notice? Did it cause you to withdraw or perhaps want to avoid engaging with others? Documenting these experiences helps externalize and demystify them, making them less intimidating. Remember that the goal here is not to solve or eradicate these feelings but to acknowledge their presence and give them space. This exercise nurtures a habit of self-reflection and gradually fosters an attitude of acceptance (Nash, 2022).

## Willingness Practice

Willingness practice involves intentionally engaging in activities that might evoke emotional discomfort. This practice is about expanding your comfort zone rather than avoiding challenging situations. Start by identifying activities that align with your values but usually trigger discomfort. This could be as simple as speaking up in a meeting or as significant as starting a new hobby that involves meeting new people.

Gradually expose yourself to these activities. For instance, if public speaking causes anxiety, begin practicing in front of a mirror and then progress to speaking to a small, supportive group before addressing a larger audience. Each step should push you slightly beyond your comfort level, helping you build tolerance for discomfort over time. The key is to focus on the value-driven purpose behind the action, not just the discomfort it brings. Over time, this practice reduces avoidance behaviors and builds resilience, enabling you to engage in life despite emotional challenges fully.

## Visualization Techniques

Visualization techniques are powerful tools for cultivating peace and acceptance. Imagine your thoughts and feelings as a flowing river; see yourself sitting on the bank, watching them pass without getting swept away. This imagery helps you allow your thoughts and emotions to flow naturally without resistance or attachment.

Here's a simple visualization exercise: Find a quiet place to sit comfortably. Close your eyes and take a few deep breaths. Picture a serene river flowing steadily in front of you. Visualize each thought as a leaf floating down the stream. Some leaves might be bright and pleasant, while others may be dark and heavy. Watch each leaf pass by without trying to catch or push it away. Observe and let it continue its journey. This exercise can be particularly soothing and help you create a mental distance from distressing thoughts by allowing you to foster an attitude of nonjudgmental observation (Moore, 2019).

## *Surrender Demonstration*

The surrender demonstration emphasizes letting go of control and trusting the process. It's crucial to understand that surrender doesn't mean giving up; instead, it means releasing the need to control every aspect of your experience. To illustrate this, imagine holding a clenched fist tightly for several minutes. Feel the tension building up in your hand and arm. Now, slowly open your fist and release the tension. Notice the relief that comes with letting go.

In real-life scenarios, surrender might mean accepting uncertainty in a job search, acknowledging the limits of your influence in a relationship, or trusting your body's healing process during illness. Practicing surrender is about recognizing what you can't control and shifting your focus to what you can—your actions, reactions, and attitude. By making peace with uncertainty and relinquishing excessive control, you can move forward with greater ease and flexibility.

To foster surrender, start by identifying the areas of your life where you exert undue control. Reflect on the impact this has on your well-being. Create mantras or affirmations to remind yourself of the importance of letting go, such as "I trust the process" or "I release what I cannot control." Use these affirmations whenever you feel overwhelmed by the need to micromanage outcomes.

### **Cognitive Defusion Exercises**

We've spoken a bit about defusions and how they can be used to reduce the intensities you feel in certain moments. Cognitive defusion is a fundamental technique in ACT that helps you reduce the influence of unwanted thoughts and beliefs on your life. This technique enables you to observe your thoughts without getting entangled in them, which can ultimately help you diminish their power.

Cognitive defusion encompasses various techniques that enable you to view your thoughts impartially. Through word repetition exercises and defusion scripts, you can significantly diminish the influence of intrusive and negative thoughts. Practicing these methods consistently can improve emotional regulation and greater psychological flexibility. Embracing these following strategies fosters a healthier relationship with our internal experiences, paving the way for a more balanced and fulfilled life:

- **Word Repetition Exercise.** This practice involves repeating troublesome words or phrases aloud or mentally until they lose their emotional intensity. For example, if "failure" causes significant distress, saying it repeatedly for a minute can render the word meaningless and lessen its hold on you. This exercise demonstrates how cognitive fusion—the process of believing our thoughts—can be disrupted, thereby making it easier to manage negative self-talk.

- **Diffusion Scripts.** Defusion scripts involve guided questions that challenge the validity of negative thoughts. These scripts might include the following questions: "What's the evidence for this thought?" or "Is this thought helpful?" Engaging with such questions encourages critical thinking and provides a structured way to examine and weaken the impact of negative thoughts. This method can also be practiced through writing, allowing deeper reflection and analyses.

# Committed Action Plans

As with all the previous strategies, taking actionable steps toward reinforcing your values will make ACT successful. Once you've done the work to write down your thoughts and analyze them through journal prompts, it's time to use committed action plans to follow through with your goals. These are some ways to stay committed to your action plans through the use of the SMART goals that you learned about in an earlier chapter:

- **Practice actionable steps daily.** Daily action steps also enhance accountability. They provide a tangible way to measure your dedication and adherence to your plans. By checking off these smaller tasks, you build momentum and confidence. This process keeps you on track and helps celebrate small wins, which can boost motivation and morale. It's like building a puzzle; each piece brings you closer to completing the big picture.

- **Anticipate common obstacles.** Anticipating obstacles is another vital component of staying committed to your values. Life is unpredictable, and setbacks are inevitable. Being prepared for potential challenges allows you to navigate them more effectively. Identify barriers such as time constraints, lack of resources, or emotional stress. Think about what might hinder your progress and prepare solutions in advance. If you anticipate having a hectic schedule, plan your action steps during less busy periods.

- **Prepare emotionally.** Emotional preparation is equally important. Understand that setbacks do not signify failure but are part of the journey. Cultivate a mindset that views challenges as opportunities for growth. For example, if you miss a daily action step, instead of feeling defeated, analyze why it happened and adjust your plan accordingly. This resilience ensures that you remain steadfast in your commitment, even when faced with difficulties.

- **Find an accountability partner.** Share your goal with someone who understands the importance of mental health. Regular check-ins can remind you why you started and how far you've come. They can encourage you on tough days and celebrate your successes, keeping your motivation high. Through this structured approach of setting SMART goals, breaking them down into actionable steps, anticipating obstacles, and fostering accountability, you can empower yourself to take consistent, value-driven actions. Accountability partnerships can significantly bolster your commitment to change. Engaging with others provides external support and motivation. These partners can be friends, family members, or even professional coaches. Share your SMART goals and daily action steps with them. Discuss your progress regularly, celebrate achievements, and seek advice when encountering obstacles. Knowing that someone else is invested in your success can be incredibly motivating.

- **Plan ahead of time.** Break this down into daily action steps. Plan your weeks, scheduling exercise sessions when you are least likely to be interrupted. Anticipate obstacles such as fluctuating motivation or unexpected events. Have a backup plan, such as shorter, high-intensity workouts for hectic days. Equip yourself emotionally by accepting that some days will be more complex. Embrace flexibility without losing sight of your end goal.

With this motivated approach, you can stick to an action plan that reaps the best results. Remember that even though your circumstances may feel overwhelming, you are in control. You can make the changes that you need to make to manage the ups and downs of life.

## Journaling Prompts

To practice cognitive defusion as a strategy to promote emotional regulation, you can answer the following prompts, which will help you accept your intense emotions while moving forward in a more positive light:

Examine a time when you felt disconnected from your values. What triggered this disconnection? Explore how it affected your mood and decisions. How can you realign with your values moving forward?

Write about a personal challenge you want to commit to changing. What steps can you take to address this challenge? Outline a plan that accepts the situation while committing to growth.

Think about an experience that brought you joy. What were the circumstances? How can you create more opportunities for joy in your life? Write a list of activities or moments you want to prioritize.

Consider how past experiences shape your current beliefs. Reflect on a significant event that impacted you. What beliefs arose from that experience? Are they still serving you well, or must they be reevaluated?

Write about a time when you practiced self-compassion. How did it change your perspective? What can you do to cultivate self-compassion more regularly?

Reflect on how you respond to criticism. What emotions do you feel upon receiving criticism? Write down your initial reaction and how you might change your response to be kinder to yourself.

Describe a situation that requires you to accept uncertainty. What feelings arise when you face the unknown? Explore ways to find peace in uncertainty and ways in which you can develop resilience.

Write about a commitment you made in the past that you're proud of. How did you stay dedicated to it? What did you learn about yourself through that commitment?

Reflect on moments of doubt. What triggers your self-doubt? Write about how you can challenge these thoughts and embrace confidence. What affirmations can you use to combat doubt?

Consider the importance of forgiveness in your life. Who do you need to forgive, including yourself? Write down your thoughts on the healing power of forgiveness and how it relates to acceptance.

Examine your daily routines. Are they aligned with your values? Write about changes you can make to ensure your days reflect who you are and what you strive for.

Finally, think about your legacy. How do you want to be remembered? Write a short paragraph capturing what you want to contribute to the world and how acceptance and commitment play a role in that vision.

# Final Thoughts on ACT Techniques

This chapter has provided practical exercises to seamlessly integrate ACT strategies into your daily life. By exploring various mindfulness practices—mindful breathing, body scan meditation, mindful eating, and walking meditation—you can develop a deeper connection to your thoughts and emotions. These exercises are designed to help you become more present, reduce stress, and embrace your emotions without experiencing any guilt about your feelings.

By consistently applying these techniques, you'll find it easier to align your actions with your values. Engaging in acceptance and willingness exercises will prepare you with the tools you need to confidently address life's challenges more effectively. Remember that the goal is not to eliminate negative thoughts or feelings but to build resilience and live a life that genuinely reflects what matters most to you.

Now that you know three great therapeutic strategies that can help you regulate your

emotions better, it's time to take a deeper dive into our bodies and understand how they function emotionally. In the following chapter, we will unpack how the vagus nerve has a direct impact on your emotions.

# Ready to live a life that aligns with your deepest values?

As a bonus, we've included a values and commitment worksheet, based on the powerful ACT framework, to help you on your journey. This worksheet will guide you in identifying your core values and aligning your actions with what truly matters. It's a powerful tool to gain clarity, make meaningful choices, and live a life that resonates with your deepest self.

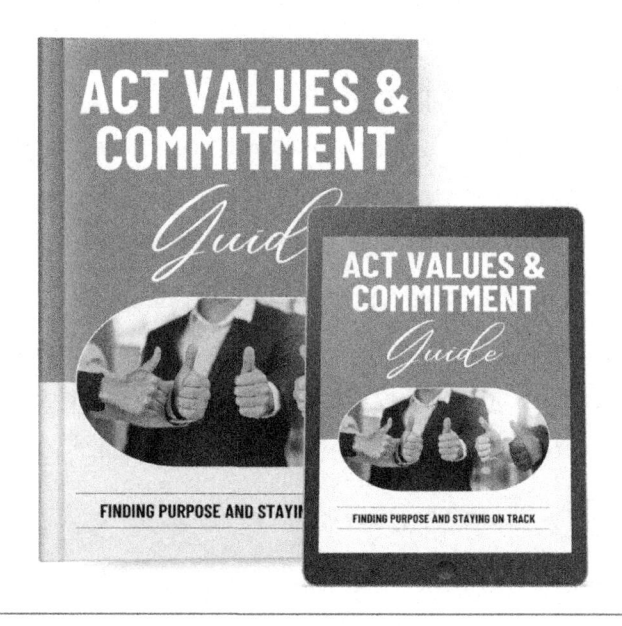

*Scan the QR Code to download your free copy now and take the first step towards a life that reflects your true priorities!*

# Chapter 7: Understanding the Vagus Nerve

Sometimes, you do all the mental work to enhance your emotional regulation. Still, you must remember the physical elements within your nervous system that impact how you manage different stimuli. Understanding the vagus nerve begins with acknowledging its role in your body. Known as "the body's superhighway," this nerve is one of the longest and most complex nerves, stretching from the brainstem down to various organs in the thorax and abdomen. It helps to link your emotional state to your physical health. The vagus nerve's extensive reach allows it to influence several crucial bodily functions, including heart rate, digestion, and respiratory rate, which are essential to maintaining homeostasis and overall well-being.

This chapter covers the fascinating anatomy and function of the vagus nerve, showcasing how it connects your emotional experiences and physical responses. You will learn about its origins, pathways, and significant tasks within both the sensory and motor systems. We will also explore how the vagus nerve facilitates the rest-and-digest activities of the parasympathetic nervous system, helping you return to a state of calm after stress. When you understand the intricate workings of this nerve, you'll gain valuable information about the techniques for managing stress and promoting relaxation, which will empower you to take control of your emotional health and improve your quality of life.

# The Anatomy and Functioning of the Vagus Nerve

The vagus nerve is the longest cranial nerve in the body. Its name is derived from the Latin word for "wanderer," because it has an extensive reach throughout the body. Emerging from the brainstem's medulla oblongata, it branches out from the neck down to various organs in the thorax and abdomen. This network helps bridge the gap between your emotional experiences and physical health.

Understanding the structure of this fascinating nerve is crucial. The vagus nerve is a pair of nerves on each side of the body. These nerves contain sensory (afferent) and motor (efferent) fibers, with approximately 80% being afferent. This means that the vagus nerve sends sensory information from the body's organs to the brain. This sensory feedback is vital for maintaining homeostasis and ensuring the body's internal environment remains stable.

You may wonder why the vagus nerve is so vital in emotional health. The answer lies in its role within the parasympathetic nervous system, responsible for the body's rest-and- digest activities. When you experience stress or danger, your sympathetic nervous system kicks into gear, triggering the fight-or-flight response. In contrast, your parasympathetic system, facilitated by the vagus nerve, helps restore calm and balance once the threat has passed.

The vagus nerve's influence on heart rate, digestion, and respiratory rate is prominent, so boosting vagal tone is crucial. For instance, when activated, the vagus nerve releases acetylcholine, a neurotransmitter that slows down the heart rate. This vagal tone, or the activity of the vagus nerve, is a marker of how well the parasympathetic nervous system is functioning. A higher vagal tone is associated with better emotional regulation and resilience, making it easier to manage stress and recover from emotional upheavals. A healthy heart rate influences several mental and physical responses, reducing anxiety and countless health issues.

The vagus nerve's impact extends to several other bodily functions besides your heart rate, digestion, and respiratory function. It affects voice modulation, swallowing, and even immune response. Sensory information from the skin of the ear, muscles involved in swallowing and speaking, and various internal organs are all processed by the vagus nerve. This broad role emphasizes the importance of maintaining overall wellness and emotional stability.

Understanding this intricate system can be empowering. It offers practical tools for managing anxiety, depression, and other emotional challenges. Techniques such as deep breathing, meditation, yoga, and cold exposure can stimulate the vagus nerve, enhancing its ability to maintain balance and promote relaxation. Practicing these techniques regularly can improve vagal tone and emotional and physical health over time.

## Polyvagal Theory Basics

Polyvagal theory, introduced by Dr. Stephen Porges, explains the relationship between your autonomic nervous system and emotional regulation abilities. This theory showcases why you respond to stress and social interactions in particular ways, emphasizing the importance of achieving a balanced state for emotional well-being.

### Understanding Neuroception

At the heart of polyvagal theory is the concept of neuroception.

Neuroception is an automatic process caused by your nervous system scanning the environment for safety or danger cues. Unlike perception, which involves conscious thought, neuroception operates below our awareness. It assesses risk and prompts your body to respond accordingly. For instance, when walking down a dimly lit street, you might feel uneasy even if nothing alarming is immediately visible. This feeling stems from neuroception, which detects potential threats based on subtle environmental cues.

Understanding neuroception can help you recognize why you may feel anxious or uncomfortable in certain situations without an apparent reason. Imagine attending a crowded party where you suddenly feel tense and want to leave. Even with no obvious danger, your neuroception may have picked up on factors such as loud noises or unfamiliar faces, triggering a stress response. These reactions are not always logical but are deeply rooted in our survival instincts.

Neuroception influences three primary states of autonomic arousal: social engagement, mobilization, and immobilization. Each of these states corresponds to different emotional responses based on perceived levels of safety or danger. The social engagement state is activated when you feel safe. In this state, you can connect with others, make eye contact, and communicate effectively. Your body remains calm, promoting prosocial behaviors and enabling you to form bonds and navigate complex social environments.

## *Considering Mobilization*

In contrast, the mobilization state kicks in when a threat is detected. This state is characterized by the "fight or flight" response, where your heart rate increases, your muscles tense up, and you prepare to confront or escape the danger.

While this reaction is crucial for survival, it can be maladaptive when triggered in nonthreatening situations. An example would be experiencing anxiety during a job interview. Despite the absence of physical danger, your body may react as if it's under threat due to the pressure and stress of the situation.

Lastly, immobilization occurs when the body perceives an overwhelming threat that cannot be escaped or fought off. This state is often associated with the freeze response. You may shut down, becoming numb and unresponsive. Think of a deer caught in headlights; unable to run or fight, it freezes. In humans, this state can manifest during traumatic events or intense fear, it leads to feelings of helplessness and dissociation.

## Its Role in Emotional Health

Achieving a regulated state is crucial for emotional well-being. When balanced, you're better equipped to handle stress and maintain effective social connections. According to polyvagal theory, your capacity to move fluidly between these states—without getting stuck in mobilization or immobilization—defines resilience and emotional health.

To foster this flexibility, polyvagal theory emphasizes the vagus nerve's role, particularly its influence on the parasympathetic nervous system. The vagus nerve acts like a brake, slowing the heart rate and promoting relaxation. Practices that stimulate the vagus nerve, such as deep breathing, mindfulness, and social engagement, can help you return to calm after experiencing stress.

Consider diaphragmatic breathing. Focusing on slow, deep breaths activates the vagus nerve, which helps reduce your heart rate and lower your stress hormones. Over time, incorporating such practices into daily routines can enhance your ability to manage anxiety and improve overall emotional resilience.

Understanding the implications of polyvagal theory extends beyond individual practices. It also sheds light on broader social dynamics. For instance, people with a heightened sensitivity to threat cues might struggle more in environments perceived as unsafe, impacting their ability to engage socially. Conversely, creating supportive and secure environments can facilitate better social interactions and emotional regulation.

Mental health practitioners can leverage these insights to support their clients more effectively. By recognizing the signs of different autonomic states, therapists can tailor interventions to help clients transition from states of mobilization or immobilization back to social engagement. Techniques such as safe touch, soothing voices, and fostering a sense of connection can play pivotal roles in this process.

## Vagus Nerve Stimulation Practices

When managing stress and promoting emotional regulation, understanding how to stimulate the vagus nerve can be a game-changer. The vagus nerve greatly influences the parasympathetic nervous system, which helps calm the body and mind, so if you can master your vagus nerve, you can effectively remain calm. The following practices can help you achieve healthy vagus nerve stimulation:

- **Cold exposure.** One powerful method to stimulate the vagus nerve is cold exposure. Exposing your body to acute cold conditions, such as taking a cold shower or splashing cold water on your face, enhances vagal tone by increasing parasympathetic activity while decreasing sympathetic activity (*How to Stimulate the Vagus Nerve*, n.d.). For beginners, start with a 30-second cold shower followed by warm water. Gradually extend the duration as your body acclimates. Once you feel comfortable with cold showers, you can explore more intense versions of cold exposure, such as ice baths. This process invigorates your body and helps bring a sense of calm and balance into your daily routine.

- **Engage your throat muscles.** Beyond physical practices, engaging in activities that involve the muscles of the throat can also boost vagal tone. Singing, humming, and gargling are simple yet effective techniques. These activities stimulate the muscles in the back of the throat, which are connected to the vagus nerve, thereby promoting feelings of well-being and relaxation. Humming, in particular, creates powerful vibrations in the nasal cavity that increase the production of nasal nitric oxide, an element known to have calming effects on the body (*How to Stimulate the Vagus Nerve*, n.d.).

- **Practice meditation.** Meditation is also an essential tool for stimulating the vagus nerve. Meditation practices help ground you in the present moment, slow down breathing, and increase emotional awareness (Harmony, 2021). Straightforward meditation practice involves sitting quietly and focusing on your breath. Notice each inhalation and exhalation without trying to change them. When your mind wanders, gently bring your focus back to your breath. Regular meditation can enhance heart rate variability, a key indicator of vagal tone, improving emotional regulation throughout the day.

- **Prioritize daily practice.** Incorporating these techniques into daily life doesn't require extensive time or effort, making them accessible for anyone looking to improve their emotional health. Small lifestyle changes can yield profound impacts. For example, starting your morning with a few minutes of deep breathing sets a relaxing tone for the day. Taking short breaks at work to splash cold water on your face can refresh your mind and reduce stress.

### How to Take Your Vagus Nerve Health to the Next Level

Understanding these techniques' simplicity empowers you to control your emotional well-being. It's comforting to know that complex technology or expensive treatments aren't necessary for significant improvements; you must consistently look after your health and well-being. Making these practices a part of your daily routine can gradually enhance your vagal tone, leading to better stress management and emotional resilience.

If you're interested in tracking progress, using a home heart rate variability (HRV) tracker with breathing exercises can offer valuable insights into vagal tone. Effective devices may be found in the higher-end price range, such as the Lief Therapeutics wearable ECG or the Polar H10 Chest Strap with the Elite HRV app (*How to Stimulate the Vagus Nerve*, n.d.). These tools can help you monitor how different practices impact your HRV and inform adjustments to your routine as needed.

Building positive social connections also contributes to enhanced vagal tone. Positive interactions, whether by spending quality time with loved ones or engaging in acts of kindness, trigger the release of oxytocin, a hormone that fosters social bonding and relaxes the body (Harmony, 2021). Even self-generated positive emotions, like those from loving-kindness meditation, where you send out positive feelings and thoughts to people in your life, can boost vagal activation and improve your sense of well-being.

Laughter is always the best medicine, and it's completely free! When you laugh, it activates a cadence of breathing that transitions the body into parasympathetic mode, enhancing vagal tone and increasing HRV. Studies show that laughter provides immediate well- being and reduces long-term anxiety (Harmony, 2021). Adding humor to your life through comedies, funny books, or spending time with friends who make you laugh can be a joyful way to support your emotional health.

Hugging and physical touch also play roles in stimulating the vagus nerve, and giving and receiving hugs releases oxytocin, further activating the parasympathetic nervous system and promoting relaxation. Such simple gestures as holding hands or being patted on the back can lower stress levels and build a sense of security and connection.

## *Loving-Kindness Meditation*

Loving-kindness is a meditative practice that you can regularly engage in to boost your happy hormones and improve your vagal tone. Here's an exercise in loving-kindness meditation that you can practice feeling more positive:

1. Find a quiet space where you can sit comfortably. Close your eyes and take a deep breath. As you inhale, imagine bringing in light and warmth. With each exhale, let go of tension and stress. Focus on your breath, feeling it flow in and out. Allow your mind to settle.

2. Now, think of someone you care about deeply. Picture their faces and think of the joy they bring into your life. Hold onto that image. Feel a warmth spreading through your chest as you think about your love for them. Let this feeling grow. With each breath, imagine sending that love to them.

3. Next, expand your thoughts to include others. Picture your friends and family, those who are close to you. Imagine the happiness and support they provide. With every inhale, draw in positive thoughts about them. With every exhale, express your gratitude. Feel each person's energy connecting with yours.

4. Then, widen your focus to include people you see regularly. The barista who makes your coffee, the neighbor who smiles at you, and even strangers in your community. Picture their faces or imagine them in your thoughts. Send good wishes to them. Think about their happiness and well-being. Let it fill your heart.

5. Now, focus on kindness. Think about small acts of kindness you can offer. A smile, a helping hand, or even a compliment. With each breath, commit yourself to practicing these acts. Imagine

how they can change someone's day. Know that your small efforts matter.

6. Begin to visualize a circle of light around you. This light represents love and positivity. As you sit in this space, allow the light to expand until it surrounds all those you visualize. See how it connects you all. Feel the warmth of community and love. Each breath strengthens this connection.

7. Consider any problematic relationships in your life. Bring those individuals to mind. Instead of anger or resentment, think about sending them love. This doesn't mean you excuse hurtful behavior but that you choose to release the weight of those feelings. Let love guide your thoughts and actions. As you continue to breathe, repeat simple phrases in your mind. "I wish that you find happiness." "I wish that you find peace." Feel the power of these words. Let them resonate in your heart. Each repetition builds compassion, both for yourself and for others.

8. In this meditation, allow yourself to feel your worthiness to receive love. You deserve kindness and happiness. Picture that loves flowing toward you. Breathe it slowly. Let it fill every space inside you. Hold onto this feeling as you move forward in your life.

9. Start to note how you feel. A sense of calmness might wash over you. You may notice a lightness in your heart. Hold onto this feeling as you prepare to bring your awareness back to the room. Wiggle your fingers and toes. Gently open your eyes when you're ready.

10. Take a moment to write down any feelings or thoughts that emerged during your meditation. Reflect on what you can do differently in your interactions. Set an intention for your day that includes showing love and kindness. Commit to carrying this energy with you as you move through the world.

11. Keep this practice in mind as you engage with others throughout your day. Each encounter is an opportunity to spread positivity. It takes little effort to express warmth with a kind word or smile. Even a brief moment of connection can brighten someone else's day.

12. Remember that this practice is not just a one-time exercise. Make it a routine. Set aside time each day or week to meditate and send out love. The more you practice, the stronger your connections will become. You'll find that love and kindness come back to you in unexpected ways.

13. Consider sharing this practice with others. Encourage friends or family to join you. Create a group meditation session focused on love and kindness. Watching others connect through this shared experience can deepen your sense of community.

14. Be mindful of your environment. Surround yourself with reminders of love. Photos of family, inspiring quotes, and even simple decorations can boost your mood. These positive influences in your space can uplift you and help maintain your intention.

15. Engage in activities that make you feel grateful. Volunteer your time, help those in need, or listen to someone who wants to share. These actions create ripples of kindness that can touch many others. Each small moment contributes to the bigger picture of love in your life.

16. When challenges arise, revisit your meditation. Return to that image of sending love. It helps you regain focus. Whenever negativity creeps in, breathe deeply and reaffirm your intention to nurture love. Let it replace any feelings of frustration.

17. Recognize the significance of self-love. Practicing kindness toward yourself is essential. Celebrate your strengths and forgive yourself for your mistakes. Treating yourself with compassion

creates a solid foundation for extending love and kindness to others.

18. Soon, you may notice that your atmosphere has changed. People will feel drawn to your positive energy. They may respond with warmth and kindness as well. Building a culture of love starts with you. Encourage others to adopt similar practices.

19. Embrace each moment as an opportunity for kindness. Consider how you can incorporate positivity, whether during mundane tasks or when making significant choices. Living with intention transforms how you experience life.

20. Let meditation practice follow you into your daily activities. Create little rituals throughout the day—pause before your meals to express gratitude, take a moment to breathe deeply in stressful situations, or give compliments freely. These simple actions make a difference.

Over time, observe the changes in your relationships. You may deepen connections and mend broken ones. Trust will increase, and joy will flourish in these bonds. Love will become a natural part of your interactions. Continue to celebrate every step in your journey toward love and kindness. Each experience, whether challenging or uplifting, will enrich your understanding. Remember that this practice is about embracing humanity and fostering connections inside and outside yourself.

## Breathing Exercises to Activate the Vagus Nerve

Apart from the exercises mentioned in the previous section, practicing breathing techniques can be a powerful way to manage your anxiety and enhance your emotional well-being by stimulating the vagus nerve.

Among these techniques, diaphragmatic breathing stands out for its simplicity and effectiveness. It focuses on altering breathing patterns to achieve a state of calm, which, in turn, impacts the vagus nerve. This method, also known as "belly breathing," involves deep inhalation through the nose, allowing the abdomen to rise, followed by a slow exhalation through the mouth. It's a deliberate way of breathing that engages the diaphragm and promotes relaxation.

The physiological processes activated by deep, controlled breathing is fascinating and motivating for those looking to adapt it into their daily routine. When you breathe deeply using your diaphragm, it signals the vagus nerve, which, in turn, activates the parasympathetic nervous system. This system is responsible for the "rest and digest" functions of the body, countering the "fight or flight" response triggered by stress. As a result, the heart rate slows, blood pressure decreases, and tension dissipates. Understanding these mechanisms can be incredibly empowering for individuals struggling with anxiety or stress, because it provides a tangible method to regain control over their emotional state. To practice diaphragmatic breathing, you can follow these steps:

1. Find a comfortable seated position and place one hand on your ribs.
2. Breathe deeply through your nose, feeling your ribs expand and your belly rise.
3. Exhale slowly through your mouth, noticing your ribs moving inward and your belly falling.
4. Repeat this for several minutes, focusing on the sensation of your breath moving in and out of your body.
5. Incorporating this into your daily routine can lead to long-term benefits in emotional regulation and overall well-being.

Another effective technique is alternate nostril breathing, which balances the nervous system and highlights the interconnectedness of your breath and emotional state. Alternate nostril breathing, or *Nadi Shodhana*, is a yogic practice done by alternating each nostril's blockage while breathing. This technique calms the mind and balances the energy channels within your body, thus promoting a sense of equilibrium and stability. The following guide can help you explore this breathing technique successfully:

1. Sit comfortably and use your right hand to close your right nostril with your thumb.

2. Inhale deeply through your left nostril, then close it with your ring and pinky fingers, and exhale through your right nostril. Inhale through your right nostril, close it, and then exhale through your left nostril.

3. Continue this pattern for several minutes, ensuring your breath is smooth and even. Regular practice can help lower stress levels, improve respiratory endurance, and reduce heart rate, improving cardiovascular health and overall well-being (Cronkleton & Walters, 2022).

Research supports the numerous benefits of alternate nostril breathing. For example, a study found that individuals who practiced this technique for 30 minutes daily experienced significantly lower perceived stress levels after three months than those who did not engage in breathing exercises. Another study demonstrated improvements in pulse and blood pressure biomarkers among participants who practiced alternate nostril breathing for four weeks, indicating potential benefits for cardiovascular health (Cronkleton & Walters, 2022).

Although both breathing techniques are great options, you should still feel inspired to research different breathing techniques to discover what works best for you. While diaphragmatic breathing and alternate nostril breathing are excellent starting points, many other practices are worth exploring, so don't limit yourself! Techniques such as box breathing, where you breathe in a pattern of four counts—inhale for four counts, hold your breath for four counts, exhale for four counts, and hold your breath again for four counts—can also be beneficial.

Navy SEALs use box breathing to remain calm under pressure. It is also valuable, because it helps regulate breathing patterns, increases mindfulness, and enhances focus. Practicing different methods allows you to develop specific approaches that meet your needs and preferences in different circumstances, making it easier to incorporate these practices into daily life.

## Impacts on Stress and Relaxation Responses

A high vagal tone correlates with enhanced emotional regulation, showing that strengthening your vagus nerve can directly influence and reduce stress levels. Understanding this connection is crucial when you're looking to improve your mental health and emotional stability. When your vagal tone is high, your body is more adept at handling stress, which benefits mental and emotional well-being. Research shows that individuals with higher vagal tone exhibit increased resilience, improved cognitive performance, and better emotional regulation (Spencer-Thomas, 2023). This means that they are better equipped to manage the daily stresses of life, whether those coming from work, personal relationships, or unexpected challenges. If you practice techniques to improve your vagal tone, you can stay calm during a heated argument or recover quickly from a stressful day at work. This ability to bounce back and maintain emotional stability is a telltale sign of good mental health.

Engaging the vagus nerve triggers a relaxation response, which aids emotional recovery and resilience. The parasympathetic nervous system, activated by the vagus nerve, promotes relaxation and enables the body to rest and digest. This process is the opposite of the fight-or-flight response triggered by the sympathetic nervous system.

When the vagus nerve is engaged, it helps slow your heart rate, decrease blood pressure, and promote a sense of calm. These physiological changes are essential for recovering from stress and building emotional resilience.

It's also helpful to understand that lifestyle choices can positively impact vagal tone. Regular physical activity, especially exercises that you enjoy, improves vagal tone and overall emotional well-being. Bodily exercise boosts cardiovascular health, stimulates the vagus nerve, and helps enhance its function.

Maintaining strong social connections is another critical factor. Engaging in positive social interactions can stimulate the vagus nerve, promoting feelings of happiness and relaxation. Spending time with friends and family, participating in group activities, and cultivating meaningful relationships can all contribute to better emotional health by enhancing vagal tone. (Bay, 2023)

This connection between the vagus nerve and emotional resilience provides a tangible goal for managing anxiety and stress in daily life. By focusing on strategies that improve vagal tone, you can work toward achieving better emotional regulation and overall mental health. For instance, incorporating daily practices—deep breathing exercises, mindfulness meditation, regular physical activity—and fostering solid social bonds can significantly impact your ability to manage stress and enhance emotional resilience.

You are in control of your vagus nerve and its condition. It's not just about managing symptoms; it's about creating an environment within the body that supports emotional stability and resilience. For example, adopting a healthy diet rich in nutrients that support brain and nervous system health can further enhance vagal tone. Foods high in omega-3 fatty acids, such as fish and flaxseeds, have been linked to improved vagal function and reduced anxiety. Similarly, adequate sleep is vital in maintaining a healthy vagal tone. Ensuring sufficient rest each night allows the body to repair and regenerate, supporting overall well-being.

Remember the importance of your self-care routines, which are key to minimizing stress and boosting overall happiness and well-being. Regularly engaging in activities that promote relaxation, and well-being can lead to lasting improvements in emotional health.

Starting small can make a big difference for those new to these concepts. Even spending 5 minutes each day practicing deep breathing or mindfulness can have profound effects over time. Consistency is critical, and the benefits will accumulate, leading to better stress management and enhanced emotional resilience.

Understanding the vagus nerve's influence on stress management and relaxation empowers you to take control of your emotional health. By focusing on practices that improve vagal tone, you can develop a more resilient and balanced approach to handling life's stresses. The knowledge that you can actively engage your body's natural relaxation mechanisms provides hope and a clear path forward if you are seeking to improve your mental health. Whether through deep breathing, mindfulness, physical activity, social connections, or a combination of these strategies, enhancing vagal tone offers a practical and effective way to manage anxiety and promote emotional well-being.

## *Journaling Prompts*

Feeling overly stressed and overwhelmed can have a drastic impact on your vagal tone, as well as your overall health. The following journal prompts can help you reduce your stress and anxiety to enhance your vagal tone:

What are three things that made you smile today? Focus on those moments and write about how they felt. Recognizing positivity, even in small doses, can help counterbalance stress.

Please describe what happened, who was involved, and why it made you smile.

Think about a challenge you faced recently. How did you handle it? Write about your feelings during that time and how you overcame the situation. Consider what you learned from this experience and how it changed your perspective. Reflect on the strengths you discovered within yourself.

Imagine a place where you feel completely at ease. It could be an actual location or a made-up one. Describe this place in detail. What do you see, hear, and feel? Write about how being in this setting affects your stress levels and what you can do to bring some elements of that place into your daily life.

What is one thing you are grateful for today? Write about it and explore why it matters to you. Reflect on how this gratitude can shift your mindset and help alleviate anxiety. Consider how gratitude practices can improve your overall well-being.

Create a list of three things you want to let go of. These could be negative thoughts, habits, or situations that cause you stress. Write about why you want to release each and what positive changes you hope to see.

Write about activities that help you recharge and reduce stress. Be specific about how these activities make you feel and how often you engage. Consider ways to prioritize self-care in your routine more consistently.

# Final Insights on the Vagus Nerve

In this chapter, you've learned about the remarkable role of the vagus nerve in emotional regulation and stress management. By understanding its extensive network within our bodies, we can see how it acts as a bridge between our emotional and physical health. The vagus nerve's ability to lower heart rate, stimulate digestion, and promote relaxation is essential in maintaining overall well-being. Techniques such as deep breathing, meditation, and cold exposure enhance vagal tone, helping you manage stress more effectively and improve your emotional resilience.

As we move forward, it's essential to incorporate these practical tools into our daily lives. Engaging the vagus nerve through simple practices can profoundly affect mental and physical health. Whether you're dealing with anxiety or depression or simply looking to build better emotional habits, understanding and utilizing the power of the vagus nerve offers a tangible way to balance those nerves. Remember that small steps can lead to significant improvements, so start incorporating these practices today and experience the benefits for yourself.

As truly as your internal well-being affects your emotional health, so does the well-being of your entire physical body. The mind–body connection is powerful and can be hacked through somatic therapy, which we will explore in detail in the next chapter.

# Feeling overwhelmed by stress and anxiety? You're not alone.

As a bonus, we've included a practical guide to help you harness the power of your vagus nerve, a key player in calming your nervous system and regulating your emotions. It's packed with easy-to-follow exercises and somatic practices you can incorporate into your daily life to manage stress, reduce anxiety, and find a greater sense of balance.

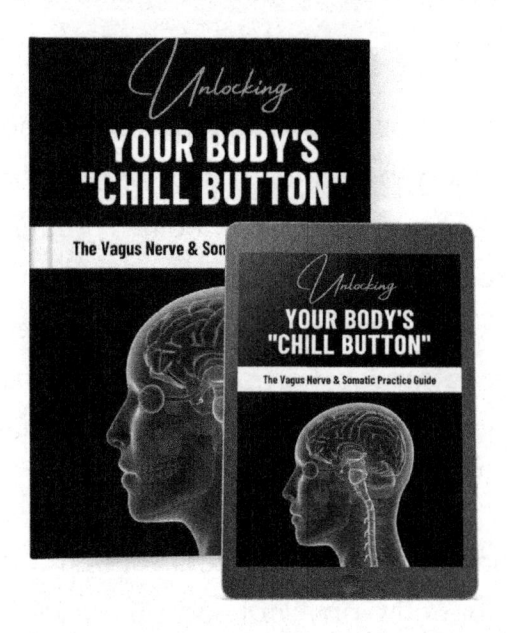

*Ready to take control of your well-being? Simply scan the QR Code to download your free copy now and start experiencing the calming power of your vagus nerve!*

# Chapter 8: Somatic Practices for Emotional Well- Being

As we move on to talking about your physical well-being and emphasizing its connection with your emotional health, let's take a look at some somatic practices. Incorporating somatic practices into your daily life provides a unique and effective way to enhance your health and happiness. By focusing on your body's role in storing and processing emotions, these techniques offer practical tools for achieving better mental health. Many people may need to know how deeply interconnected their physical sensations and emotional states are and how addressing one can positively impact the other. Whether it's through simple exercises or more structured therapeutic methods, somatic practices open new pathways for understanding and managing your emotional worlds.

This chapter will explore various somatic techniques that can be seamlessly integrated into your everyday routines. You'll learn the critical concepts of somatic experiencing (SE), emphasizing body awareness and grounding as essential emotional regulation tools. You'll also discover specific methods such as progressive muscle relaxation (PMR), mindful breathing, and the power of embracing nature to enhance your sensory experiences. Through situational examples and practical exercises, this chapter will equip you with actionable strategies to strengthen your connection between your body and mind, ultimately leading to improved emotional health.

# Basics of SE

When it comes to emotional health and well-being, recognizing the role of the body in the system of thoughts and feelings is crucial. Incorporating SE into daily routines can unlock pathways to better mental health by focusing on how our bodies store and process emotions. Here, we aim to introduce you to the foundational concepts of SE and demonstrate its relevance to emotional health.

### SE: Understanding the Body's Role in Healing

SE is a therapeutic method designed to help people recover from the trauma and stress stored in their bodies. Unlike other therapies that focus primarily on thoughts or feelings, SE highlights how the body can be a path to recovery. The idea behind SE is that trauma impacts not just our minds but also our entire nervous system. This can lead to various physical and emotional issues if not adequately addressed.

It is essential to recognize that our bodies can hold emotional memories. Everyone has experienced situations where they felt physical reactions to stress, like having *butterflies* in their stomach or feeling a tightness in their chest during tough times. These bodily sensations are real and show how closely linked our emotions and physical sensations are. When you face trauma or considerable stress, your body may store these experiences. This storage can sometimes lead to an ongoing imbalance in your nervous system, resulting in emotional and physical symptoms that may linger long after the event. The following are some critical factors of somatic therapy that make it an effective practice:

- **Body awareness.** One of the key ideas in somatic therapies is improving body awareness, which means being aware of what you feel physically and understanding how those sensations link to your emotions. For example, when someone feels tension in their shoulders, recognizing that feeling may reveal it is tied to stress.

Grounding techniques are vital aspects of SE that help people stay connected to the present moment, promoting stability. For instance, grounding might involve noticing how your feet feel against the ground. These practices form the foundation of SE therapy.

- **Sense of safety.** A crucial part of SE is creating a sense of safety. Many trauma survivors find it challenging to feel secure in their bodies. Establishing a safe physical and mental environment is the first step in therapy. This might start with simple actions that build trust, such as being mindful of bodily sensations in a calm setting. Over time, as an individual becomes more comfortable, they may be able to explore and release the energy that has been trapped in their bodies due to trauma. This process can lead to a reduction in symptoms such as anxiety or chronic pain.

- **Grounding techniques.** Grounding techniques can be helpful tools for reconnecting with the present. Simple practices such as feeling the ground beneath your feet or touching the fabric of your clothes can enhance this connection. Regularly practicing grounding can ease overwhelming feelings and help people feel more secure. This sense of safety is crucial for emotional regulation and helps individuals better manage their feelings.

- **Pendulation.** Another exciting aspect of SE is the idea of "pendulation." Pendulation is about the natural shift between feelings of discomfort and comfort. This allows individuals to explore distressing memories without feeling completely overwhelmed. By moving back and forth between challenging sensations and feelings of safety, individuals can start to process and integrate their experiences. This balance respects the body's natural healing process and ensures that therapeutic progress occurs appropriately for the individual.

Think about a war veteran dealing with post-traumatic stress disorder. Traditional talk therapy may not always capture the full extent of the effects of their trauma. However, integrating SE into their treatment could allow them to explore their memories of combat more effectively. Using gentle exercises that highlight bodily sensations, the veteran can release the survival energy that remained trapped in their body during traumatic events. The same can be said for any traumatic experience.

Engaging in SE is a complex but rewarding journey. It takes time, self-compassion, and a willingness to explore the profound connection between your body and mind. SE offers a valuable path for those struggling with anxiety, depression, or emotional regulation. You can start making meaningful strides toward better emotional health by focusing on your body's natural wisdom and using techniques that foster awareness and grounding.

## Tracking and Grounding Practices

Understanding and harnessing the power of bodily awareness can be a transformative practice for improving emotional well-being. By providing practical techniques for tracking bodily sensations and grounding yourself in the present moment, you can better manage your stress and anxiety symptoms. The following points can help you ground yourself when you're feeling overwhelmed.

- **Become aware of sensations.** One of the fundamental steps in somatic practices involves becoming aware of and identifying different sensations experienced in various body parts. This process starts by paying attention to physical cues such as tightness, warmth, tingling, or other subtle feelings that arise. For example, you might notice tension in your shoulders when stressed or fluttering sensation in your stomach when anxious. By regularly tuning into these signals, you can begin to associate specific emotions with particular bodily sensations. Distinguishing between sensations is also crucial. A feeling of heaviness might indicate fatigue, while a light buzzing could be related to excitement or nervousness. Developing this nuanced understanding enables more accurate self-assessments and timely interventions.

- **Embrace nature.** Nature offers a long list of benefits as a grounding tool. Spending time outdoors, whether walking in a park or gardening, can significantly enhance emotional well-being. Nature immersion provides a break from technology and daily stressors, allowing you to reconnect with your natural environment. Practical ways to incorporate nature into your routine include taking a mindful walk, where you focus on the sights, sounds, and smells around you. Feel the texture of leaves, listen to the chirping sounds of birds, and notice the fresh scent of grass or flowers. Gardening is another excellent way to ground yourself; handling soil, planting seeds, and tending to plants engage multiple senses and create a sense of accomplishment. Even if access to green spaces is limited, bringing elements of nature indoors, such as houseplants or natural materials, can provide similar calming effects.

- **Find a personalized grounding technique.** Establishing a customized grounding routine that integrates seamlessly into daily life is essential for sustained emotional well-being. Start by identifying activities that naturally fit your schedule and appeal to your senses. For instance, begin your day with a simple grounding exercise; for example, stretching, focusing on the sensations in your muscles and joints as you move. Incorporate deep breathing exercises throughout the day; pausing to take a few mindful breaths can quickly reset your focus and reduce stress. During breaks at work, consider short walks outside or brief meditative periods where you sit quietly and tune into your surroundings.

- **Establish a bedtime routine.** Creating a bedtime ritual with grounding practices can improve sleep quality and relaxation. Techniques such as PMR, where you systematically tense and release different muscle groups, can help you release accumulated tension. Visualization exercises, where you picture a calm and safe place, can also serve as effective grounding methods before sleep. Integrating these practices consistently turns them into habitual routines that support emotional regulation.

To find what works best for you, experiment with different techniques and note which ones resonate most. Some may find that tactile activities, such as knitting or playing with a small object, provide the best grounding experience, while others might prefer auditory methods, such as listening to music or guided meditations. The key is to remain flexible and adaptable, allowing your routine to evolve as you discover what works best for you.

## Body Scans and PMR

To truly understand the power of somatic practices for emotional well-being, it's essential to explore how techniques such as body scans and PMR can facilitate emotional release and relaxation. These methods are not just about physical relaxation but also about boosting your mental health.

A body scan is a guided technique that systematically focuses awareness of different body parts. A body scan aims to help individuals become more aware of their physical presence and sensations and aid the release of tension and emotional strain. Here's how you can go about practicing this valuable exercise:

1. Begin by finding a quiet, comfortable place to lie down or sit without distractions.

2. Close your eyes and take a few deep breaths to center yourself.

3. Start at the top of your head and mentally note any sensations, tension, warmth, or discomfort.

4. Gradually move your focus downward through your face, neck, shoulders, arms, chest, abdomen, hips, legs, and feet.

5. Spend a few moments on each area, acknowledging any sensations without judgment. Observing and accepting your feelings is critical, allowing tension to dissolve naturally.

When used in tandem with body scans, PMR can offer profound benefits. PMR involves sequentially tensing and then relaxing different muscle groups throughout the body. This method reduces physical tension and enhances emotional clarity by shifting the body's physiological state from stress to relaxation.

1. To begin, settle into a comfortable position and close your eyes.
2. Take a few slow, deep breaths.Start with your toes—inhale deeply and squeeze the muscles tightly, holding the tension for about 5 seconds.
3. Then, exhale slowly, releasing the tension and noticing the feeling of relaxation.
4. Move up to your calves, thighs, buttocks, abdomen, hands, arms, shoulders, neck, jaw, and finally, your forehead, repeating the tensing and relaxing process for each muscle group.

One powerful way to harness the benefits of these techniques is by combining them. For instance, during a particularly stressful day at work, you could take a moment to do a quick body scan while seated at your desk. Notice if you're clenching your jaw or tensing your shoulders. Then, integrate PMR by consciously tensing and relaxing those areas. This combination helps in immediate stress reduction and fosters a deeper connection between mind and body, promoting long-term emotional health.

Situational examples can help you put these techniques into context. Imagine you're about to give a big presentation. Your heart races, and your muscles tighten as anxiety sets in. By doing a body scan, you identify that your shoulders are tense. You then practice PMR by tightening and releasing those shoulder muscles and following it with a few deep breaths. This quick routine shifts your body's state, calming your sympathetic nervous system and helping you regain composure. Similarly, before bedtime, a full- body scan coupled with PMR can ease you into relaxation, preparing your body for restful sleep.

If you struggle with anxiety, depression, or emotional imbalances, these two techniques can do wonders when addressing immediate emotional struggles. They create a sense of control and mindfulness that can relieve constant emotional turmoil. Body scans and PMR provide structured methods to foster change and growth for individuals interested in self-improvement. Integrating these practices into daily routines can cultivate a deeper awareness of their physical and emotional states, leading to greater emotional resilience and clarity.

To further support the development of these personalized practices, here are some guidelines:

- **Set Clear Intentions**: Before starting a session, decide your goal. Whether reducing anxiety or simply unwinding after a long day, having a clear intention helps guide your practice.
- **Find a Quiet Space**: Consistent practice in a peaceful environment minimizes distractions and enhances the effectiveness of these techniques.
- **Use Resources**: Guided recordings or apps can be beneficial, especially for beginners. Over time, you may feel confident enough to practice on your own.

- **Be Patient**: Building a new habit takes time. Keep going if you see immediate results. Consistency is key to experiencing the long-term benefits.

- **Track Your Progress**: Keeping a journal of your experiences can help you notice patterns and improvements over time, reinforcing the benefits of your practice.

## Movement-Based Therapies and Exercises

Exploring various movement-based techniques to promote emotional health and well- being can significantly enhance your mental state. Movement therapies offer a unique way to access emotions and facilitate emotional release, providing an alternative or complementary method to traditional talk therapy or medication.

Using movement for emotional regulation has profound and accessible therapeutic benefits. When you engage in physical activities such as dancing or yoga, you create opportunities for emotional catharsis. This process allows you to express and release emotions such as anger, sadness, or frustration that might remain suppressed. By physically moving through these emotions, you can find new ways to understand and manage your feelings.

Movement-based therapies come in many forms, each contributing uniquely to emotional and mental health. Here are a few movement-based therapies you can consider:

- **Yoga**, for instance, combines breath control, meditation, and poses to achieve a sense of peace and inner balance. It helps reduce stress levels, alleviate symptoms of anxiety and depression, and improve overall well-being.

- **Tai Chi**, a form of Chinese martial arts, involves slow, deliberate movements and deep breathing, which are known to modulate brain regions involved in mood regulation and reduce stress (Sani et al., 2023).

- **Dance therapy** utilizes music and spontaneous movement to facilitate self- expression and emotional release.

Each of these practices offers physical benefits and significant psychological advantages by promoting mindfulness and encouraging a deeper connection with yourself.

Practicing movement therapy doesn't necessarily require a lot of time, space, or specialized equipment. Accessible exercises can be done at home, which allows you to integrate these beneficial practices into your daily routine without much hassle. Simple yoga stretches or a few minutes of mindful breathing can make a difference. For example, starting the day with a short series of sun salutations can invigorate your body and calm your mind, setting a positive tone for what lies ahead. Similarly, a quick session of mindful walking around your home or garden can benefit physical activity and mental clarity.

Group classes can also offer social support and a sense of community. Joining a local yoga class or dance group can provide additional emotional benefits by establishing connections with others with similar interests. These social interactions can alleviate feelings of isolation and loneliness, positively affecting your emotional health. Sharing experiences and progress with a supportive group can reinforce your commitment to regular practice and amplify the therapeutic effects of movement.

It's essential to remember that movement-based therapies are highly beneficial but should be approached with an open mind and a willingness to explore. Everyone's experience will differ, and listening to your body and going at your own pace is crucial.

Here's a quick movement exercise that you can practice feeling more relaxed and positive when you need to:

1. Start by finding a comfortable spot where you can move freely. Stand up straight and keep your feet shoulder-width apart. Take a deep breath and extend your arms over your head, stretching your fingers toward the sky. Hold that stretch for a moment and feel the tension lift away. As you exhale, slowly lower your arms and let your shoulders drop. Repeat this three times to help center yourself.

2. From there, begin to rotate your shoulders. Lift them toward your ears, roll them back, and let them drop down. Do this gentle motion five times and then switch directions. These shoulder rolls release tightness and increase blood flow. Pay attention to how your body feels; this exercise opens up your upper back and neck.

3. Now, it's time to add some gentle twists. Place your hands on your hips and slowly twist your torso to the right. Hold this position briefly as you feel the stretch along your spine. Return to the center and then twist to the left. Repeat these two or three times on each side. These twists help promote flexibility and relieve tension in your back.

4. For the next movement, find a way to point at your toes. Stand tall and lift one leg, bending your knee slightly. Point your toes straight ahead, flex your foot, and stretch your toes back toward you. Alternate between pointing and flexing for each leg. Do this for about 1 minute, allowing the movement to ease leg tightness.

5. After this, let's focus on your wrists. Extend your arms in front of you, palms facing down. Rotate your wrists clockwise for thirty seconds and then switch to counterclockwise. This simple exercise helps you alleviate any stiffness, especially if you spend much time typing or holding objects. Notice how your wrists feel loose

afterward.

6. Next, find a way to incorporate some hip movements. Stand straight, keeping your feet shoulder-width apart again. Place your hands on your hips and circle with them—think hula hoop! Move in one direction for about 30 seconds and then switch to the other direction. Allow your body to relax as you engage in this fluid motion that relieves pressure and helps your hips feel more flexible.

7. Now, you can practice some light jumps. Begin with a gentle bounce on your toes, lifting your heels off the ground slightly. Keep it soft and relaxed. You can do this for about 1 minute, focusing on the rhythm of your breath. Feel the energizing effect as your heart rate rises gently, boosting your mood.

8. Let's return to some standing stretches. Extend your arms over your head and then lean to the right side, stretching your left side. Hold this momentarily, then switch to the left side to stretch your right side. Return to the center and dive forward, letting your arms dangle down toward the floor. Take a deep breath here as you release any residual tension.

9. From there, move into some gentle knee bends. Stand tall and lower your body into a partial squat. Make sure to keep your knees behind your toes and your chest lifted. Hold the squat for a few moments and then rise back up. Repeat it three to five times. This movement will help strengthen your legs while also promoting relaxation.

10. After the knee bends, let's try an easy balance exercise. Stand on one leg while bringing the other knee up to your chest. If needed, hold onto a wall or a chair for support. Hold this position for about 15 seconds before switching legs. Balancing actions like this enhances focus and stability, grounding you further in the

moment.

11. Finally, finish with a relaxation pose. Find a comfortable spot on the floor or your mat and sit cross-legged. Close your eyes and place your hands on your knees with your palms facing upward. Take a few deep breaths, letting the air fill your lungs fully. As you breathe out, let any remaining tension melt away. Visualize positive energy circulating throughout your body. Stay here for a few moments, enjoying the sense of calm and relaxation before slowly returning to your day.

You can practice these movements whenever you feel overwhelmed and stressed. They will distract you and help you release the pent-up tension and stress in your body.

# Connection Between Body and Mind Awareness

Understanding the prevalent link between bodily sensations and mental health is valuable in your journey toward emotional well-being. This interconnectedness, often called the "mind–body connection," helps you practice a more holistic approach to emotional health.

### *The Interconnectedness of Thoughts, Emotions, and Physical Sensations*

Our thoughts, emotions, and physical sensations are closely linked. The interactions between these elements greatly influence your overall well-being. For instance, when you experience stress, your body may react with physical symptoms such as headaches or muscle tension. On the other spectrum, experiencing physical ailments can lead to emotional distress. This dynamic relationship is supported by scientific research that shows us how physiological functions impact cognitive processes and vice versa (Schmitt & Schoen, 2022).

Well-known neuroscientists Damasio and Carvalho (2013) explained how sensory perturbations—misalignments between reality and our mental projections—can trigger significant cognitive attention. When our body's physical state does not align with our mental expectations, this disconnect prompts a surge in awareness, compelling us to adjust our physical or emotional state.

## Daily Practices and Feedback Loops

Enhancing the awareness of your body's cues requires daily practices that create feedback loops. These loops help you better understand and respond to your bodily sensations. One effective method is to practice mindfulness techniques such as body scanning, where you pay attention to your physical sensations from head to toe, noticing areas of tension or discomfort. Doing this allows you to identify patterns and triggers related to specific emotions, which, in turn, fosters a deeper understanding of your body's responses. Journaling can also be a reflective tool, allowing you to document physical sensations and corresponding emotional states.

Regularly checking in on your body several times daily can be incredibly beneficial. Simple questions such as "How is my body feeling right now?" or "What emotions am I experiencing?" can guide you toward better body-mind alignment. Techniques such as mindful breathing and focusing on your breath and its effect on your body can also heighten awareness and promote relaxation. These practices help bridge the gap between physical sensations and emotional responses, making it easier to manage and prevent automatic negative emotions.

## Addressing the Disconnection Brought on by Stress

Stress and adverse experiences can often lead to a disconnection between mind and body. This disconnection manifests in various ways, including numbness, chronic tension, and difficulty in identifying or expressing emotions. Reestablishing this connection requires suitable strategies that gradually restore the communication between your body and mind.

Therapeutic approaches such as mindful awareness in body-oriented therapy (MABT) are designed to address these types of disconnections. MABT combines psychoeducation and somatic techniques to scaffold interoceptive awareness, aiding you in accessing and interpreting your internal bodily signals, which is crucial for emotion regulation (Price & Hooven, 2018).

## Advocacy for Continued Practice of Body Awareness

To ensure long-term mental health benefits, you must consistently practice body awareness. It is not enough to engage occasionally; consistency is key. Regularly incorporating body awareness practices into your routine helps build resilience and a more profound connection with your emotional landscape. Over time, these practices can become second nature, providing ongoing support for managing stress and emotional challenges.

One way to ensure consistency is to integrate these practices into daily activities. For example, setting aside a few minutes each morning for mindful breathing or making it a habit to perform a quick body scan before bed can weave these routines seamlessly into your life. These few moments can do wonders for your long-term health and well-being.

Understanding and practicing body awareness allows for early detection of emotional imbalance, enabling proactive management rather than reactive coping. By staying attuned to your body, you can recognize early signs of stress or anxiety and implement calming practices before they escalate.

Creating a supportive environment that encourages body awareness can enhance these benefits. Share your practices with family or friends or find online communities prioritizing holistic health approaches. Mutual support can reinforce the importance of these practices, ensuring that they remain a consistent part of your health regimen.

## Journal Prompts

Although somatic therapy is all about your physical sensations, journaling can help you connect with your emotional side at the same time. Here are some journal prompts that can help you learn more about yourself through somatic therapy:

What physical sensations do you experience when you feel anxious? Write about the areas of your body that feel tight or uncomfortable. Explore what these sensations mean to you.

When you think of a happy memory, what feelings do you notice in your body? Describe the warmth, lightness, or any other sensations. Imagine where these feelings are located in your body.

What emotion do you struggle to express? Identify it and let your hand write down how that emotion feels physically. Is there heat, tension, or perhaps a sense of heaviness? Write freely without judgment.

Think of a time when you felt overwhelmed. What did your body do in response? Did you fidget, hold your breath, or feel lightheaded? Reflect on how these reactions relate to your emotions and thoughts during that moment.

Find a place in your body that feels safe. Describe this sensation. What does it feel like to be there? Disconnect from any noise around you and focus only on that safe feeling within your body.

What parts of your body do you avoid noticing? Write about why these areas seem disconnected. Is there pain, numbness, or maybe just indifference? Explore this disconnection and what it might represent in your life.

When was the last time you felt truly grounded? What sensations helped you connect to the earth beneath you? Write about how this connection grounds you and offers a sense of stability. Picture a stressful moment from your day. What physical sensations arose at that time? Were your hands clammy, or was there a knot in your stomach?

Reflect on how your body reacts in stressful situations and what these reveals about your coping mechanisms.

What do you feel when someone hugs you? Explore sensations of safety, warmth, or even discomfort. Write about how physical touch impacts your emotions and fosters a sense of connection or isolation in your body.

If you were to breathe into a specific area where tension resides, which location would you choose? Write about what happens to that tension as you breathe in and out. Does it dissolve, shift, or remain?

Describe your body's energy levels throughout the day. When do you feel most energetic, and when do you want to hide? Explore the connection between your physical state and your emotional well-being during these times.

What does your body need more of? Consider activities that nourish your physical being, such as movement, rest, or nutritious food.

Write about how meeting these needs can enhance your emotional health.

## Closing Remarks on Somatic Practices

In this chapter, we've journeyed through the principles and practices of SE, discovering how your body stores and processes emotions. Exploring techniques such as heightened body awareness and grounding exercises showcase the importance of being in tune with your physical sensations for enhanced mental health. Whether it's understanding how trauma manifests in your body or practicing mindful breathing to anchor yourself in the present, these methods offer practical tools for managing anxiety and depression and emotional regulation. We've also seen how addressing physical manifestations of trauma can lead to improved emotional well-being.

Creating personalized routines helps you incorporate somatic practices, emphasizing the importance of consistency and mindfulness. From performing daily body scans to using nature as a grounding tool, integrating these techniques into your life can strengthen the bond between your mind and body. Prioritize regular practice to support your growth and improve relationships. Embracing the wisdom of your body helps you pave the way toward a more balanced and emotionally resilient life. It's true when they say that you hold unhealed trauma in your body. With somatic therapy, you can start healing from all that pent-up trauma.

Another effective strategy that can be used to heal from trauma is eye movement desensitization and reprocessing, which will be discussed in the next chapter.

# Chapter 9: Eye Movement Desensitization and Reprocessing

If you've experienced past traumas that you haven't healed, then you may find it valuable to practice eye movement desensitization and reprocessing (EMDR). This chapter unravels the intricate process of EMDR, showing you how this therapeutic approach can make distressing memories less emotionally charged. Developed by psychologist Francine Shapiro in the late 1980s, EMDR leverages the brain's natural healing capabilities using a structured methodology involving eye movements or other forms of bilateral stimulation. By learning about these techniques, you can alleviate the burden of unresolved traumatic experiences, paving the way for emotional healing and resilience.

Throughout this chapter, you'll learn about the theoretical foundations and practical applications of EMDR. We'll start with an overview of how traumatic memories can impact your emotional and physical well-being and then shift to explaining how EMDR influences the integration of these memories in a more positive and healthy light. The eight phases of EMDR treatment are meticulously outlined, providing a step-by-step guide to understanding each phase's role in emotional recovery. This chapter also explores bilateral stimulation exercises, their use in daily life, and the benefits of journaling as a supplementary tool to enhance the therapy's effectiveness. Through the tips, advice, and information found in these pages, you will have a comprehensive understanding of how EMDR works, its benefits, and how it can be a powerful tool for anyone dealing with anxiety, depression, or emotional dysregulation.

## Overview of EMDR Methodology

EMDR is a therapeutic approach primarily used for trauma resolution that is now a widely respected method for facilitating the processing of distressing memories to reduce their emotional impact and promote emotional healing. The following points can enlighten you on what EMDR is and how it works as a methodology:

- **It is a grounding technique.** EMDR therapy is based on the understanding that traumatic events can leave unresolved distress within your memory. These unresolved memories can trigger emotional, psychological, and even physical. reactions when similar situations arise in the present. The core purpose of EMDR is to help you process these disturbing memories so that they become less emotionally charged and are integrated into a more adaptive knowledge base.

- **It triggers your brain's natural healing process**. EMDR therapy showcases your brain's natural ability to heal, leveraging your mind's capacity to create adaptive information processing. Through a structured eight-phase approach, EMDR facilitates this natural healing process by focusing on specific eye movements or other bilateral stimulation methods. As you recall distressing memories while experiencing bilateral stimulation, your brain integrates these experiences into a more coherent, less distressing narrative. This results in decreased emotional reactivity and increased resilience.

- **It complements alternative therapeutic practices.** Furthermore, EMDR complements other therapeutic methods by addressing the underlying emotional impacts of trauma. While CBT focuses extensively on altering dysfunctional thought patterns and behaviors, EMDR emphasizes the emotional and sensory dimensions of traumatic memories. This holistic approach ensures that both the cognitive and emotional aspects of trauma you've experienced are addressed, which leads to more comprehensive healing outcomes. Studies have shown that EMDR can be highly effective even without extensive homework, commonly required in CBT. This makes it an appealing option for individuals who may find it challenging to engage in structured daily activities due to severe trauma symptoms.

- **It encourages deeper explorations of your emotions.** A significant feature of EMDR is its ability to promote a deeper exploration of emotional wounds. Unlike some therapies that might involve gradual exposure to trauma-related content, EMDR often leads to rapid symptom relief, sometimes within just a few sessions. Clients frequently report a notable decline in distress and improved emotional regulation. This swift reduction in symptoms can be particularly beneficial for those suffering from severe post-traumatic stress disorder (PTSD) or other trauma-related conditions. Research indicates that EMDR alleviates emotional distress and improves cognitive functioning and overall well-being, promoting a proactive role in emotional healing.

- **It treats various disorders.** In addition to its efficacy with trauma, EMDR has shown promise in treating a range of psychological and somatic disorders. For example, it has been used to address anxiety, depression, phobias, and even medically unexplained physical symptoms such as chronic pain and stress-related skin conditions. EMDR's adaptability to various issues highlights its versatility as a therapeutic tool. By helping people process unresolved memories, EMDR paves the way for adaptive resolutions, thus enabling individuals to lead more fulfilling and emotionally balanced lives.

- **It has been proven successful.** The success of EMDR in fostering emotional healing is also reflected in numerous clinical trials and studies. According to Shapiro (2014), EMDR has consistently demonstrated rapid reductions in negative emotions and disturbing images associated with traumatic experiences. Further research supports the idea that EMDR can achieve treatment effects comparable to or exceeding those of traditional therapies such as CBT, often with fewer sessions and no homework requirements. This efficiency is particularly valuable for mental health practitioners with high patient loads and limited resources.

- **It is internationally recognized.** Given these advantages, EMDR is recommended by several national and international organizations as an effective treatment for PTSD and other trauma-related conditions. Its recognition by the American Psychiatric Association and the World Health Organization underscores its credibility and importance in modern psychological practice. However, it is essential for practitioners to receive specialized training in EMDR to ensure that they apply it safely and effectively, because the nuances of the approach require a thorough understanding of its principles and techniques.

For adults struggling with anxiety, depression, or emotional regulation, EMDR offers a promising avenue for addressing deep-seated emotional wounds and enhancing overall mental health. By tapping into the brain's inherent healing capacities, EMDR enables individuals to move past traumas and build resilience. As a complementary therapy, it enhances the benefits of existing treatments, providing a more rounded approach to emotional healing.

# Phases of EMDR Treatment

EMDR therapy is a structured approach that facilitates trauma recovery through eight distinct phases. Each phase builds on the previous one, creating a well-crafted pathway for emotional healing and the processing of complex trauma narratives.

### Phase 1: History Taking and Treatment Planning

The first phase, history taking and treatment planning, involves an in-depth discussion between the therapist and you. This phase lays the groundwork for a secure therapeutic relationship. The therapist carefully gathers your history, identifies traumatic events to address, and assesses both internal and external resources. This information helps you identify what will help you make progress and what pace feels comfortable for you.

### Phase 2: The Preparation Phase

In the preparation phase, the therapist educates you about the processes and expectations of EMDR therapy. Addressing any concerns or questions you may have is essential to establishing a safe therapeutic alliance. Collaboratively, you and your therapist will prepare specific coping techniques to manage any emotional disturbances that might arise during therapy. This groundwork is crucial because it helps you feel safe and ready to tackle more challenging phases of the treatment.

### Phase 3: The Assessment Phase

During the assessment phase, you will identify the event that has been suppressed, known as the "target event." This involves exploring related images, beliefs, feelings, and sensations associated with the event. Initial baseline measures are established using scales such as the subjective disturbance units and cognition validity. These measures help gauge your level of distress and the strength of your positive beliefs regarding the event.

## Phase 4: The Desensitization Phase

The desensitization phase marks the beginning of reprocessing. Using dual attention bilateral stimulation (BLS), such as side-to-side eye movements or tactile stimulation, your therapist will activate your information processing system while keeping you anchored in the present moment. This phase continues until your subjective units of disturbance rating reaches zero, indicating that the distress associated with the event has been significantly reduced.

## Phase 5: The Installation Phase

Next, the installation phase reinforces positive beliefs identified during earlier stages. Your therapist uses BLS to help you associate these positive beliefs with the reprocessed memories until they feel entirely true. Strengthening these adaptive beliefs fosters a more resilient and constructive outlook on past traumatic experiences.

## Phase 6: The Body Scan Phase

Following installation, the body scan phase aims to identify and release any residual physical tension related to the target memory. Your therapist will guide you through a mental scan of your body to detect lingering sensations or discomfort. Using BLS, any remaining disturbances are processed until you feel a sense of calm and reach a resolution.

## Phase 7: Closure

Closure is a vital part of each EMDR session, ensuring that you leave feeling safe and grounded. Your therapist will help you return to equilibrium by reviewing progress made during the session and reminding you of coping techniques. If necessary, you'll be provided with alternative strategies to reinforce your residual distress until the next EMDR session.

## Phase 8: The Reevaluation Phase

Finally, the reevaluation phase assesses the effectiveness of the previous session and determines if additional reprocessing is needed. You and your therapist will review changes in symptoms, beliefs, and emotions related to the targeted memory. This phase ensures continuity in treatment and allows for adjustments based on the client's evolving needs.

A skilled therapist plays a crucial role throughout the EMDR process. They ensure emotional safety by pacing the treatment appropriately and not rushing the emotional processing. Their expertise in navigating the intricate phases of EMDR fosters an environment where you can explore deeply rooted traumas without feeling overwhelmed.

Healing through EMDR is viewed as a journey rather than a linear process. Each phase contributes to an intricate cycle of healing, where you revisit and reprocess complex trauma narratives gradually. This progressive approach acknowledges that trauma recovery is multifaceted and requires patience and persistence.

## Journaling for EMDR Processing

Journaling, as a tool to complement EMDR, offers significant benefits by providing an additional layer of emotional support and awareness when you're undergoing therapy. By integrating journaling into the EMDR process, you can find a safe outlet for immediate expression and reflection after your therapy sessions.

### Enhancing EMDR Effectiveness with Journaling

Journaling complements EMDR by offering a dedicated outlet for expressing thoughts and emotions after sessions. Therapy often unearths intense feelings and past experiences that need further exploration. Writing provides a structured way to capture these emotions in real-time, thus enabling you to process them outside of therapy.

This immediate expression can prevent overwhelming emotions from festering, thereby reducing anxiety and enhancing overall therapeutic outcomes. Research highlights that writing about traumatic experiences helps organize your thoughts and improve emotional clarity and adaptive thinking (Siegel-Acevedo, 2021).

## Specific Journaling Prompts Tailored for EMDR Work

Prompts are crucial for guiding the journaling process, primarily when documenting emotional surges and thoughts related to trauma. Specific prompts designed for EMDR work can help you focus on the critical aspects of your healing journey. The following are examples of some prompts that you can use:

1. What emotions surfaced during today's EMDR session?
2. How did I physically feel during and after my session?
3. Which memories or images were most prominent, and why do they appear?
4. Can I identify any shifts in my perspective or emotions compared to previous sessions?
5. What self-care practices can I engage in following today's session?

These prompts help you in the process of articulating your experiences methodically, thus promoting deeper self-awareness. In addition, they offer a roadmap for capturing complex emotional landscapes, making it easier to detect patterns and shifts over time (Betterup, n.d.).

## *Alignment with EMDR's Phases*

Integrating journaling with EMDR aligns seamlessly with your therapy's structured phases. Journaling can be used to monitor progress within the eight phases discussed previously and serve as a tangible record of changes and developments. During the initial stages, journaling might focus on establishing safety and exploring the history of trauma. You can document your feelings about starting therapy and outline your goals and expectations.

As therapy progresses toward desensitization and reprocessing phases, journaling can capture your emotional reactions and cognitive shifts prompted by bilateral stimulation in real-time. Reflective entries during this stage may include descriptions of visual or auditory cues used in sessions and the emotional responses elicited. These records provide valuable feedback for the therapist and the client, making it easier to adjust therapeutic strategies based on documented experiences.

Journaling reinforces newly integrated, positive beliefs in the final phases, which involve consolidation and future planning. You can reflect on your growth, the reduction of your trauma symptoms, and your readiness to face future challenges. This written testament to progress develops a sense of accomplishment and reinforces the efficacy of EMDR therapy.

## *Long-Term Benefits of Regular EMDR-Focused Journaling*

The sustained journaling practice, centered around EMDR themes, offers numerous long-term benefits. One of the primary advantages is enhancing clarity and organization of thoughts. When emotions and thoughts are documented consistently, you find it easier to recognize patterns and track emotional growth. This process fosters a greater understanding of your deep-rooted trauma, thus empowering you to confront any overwhelming moments from your past.

Regular journaling also creates a thorough record of your healing journey, which can be incredibly validating. Revisiting past entries reveals how much progress you have made, which reinforces confidence in the therapeutic process. It serves as a reminder of resilience and survival, both essential elements for anyone recovering from trauma.

Furthermore, journaling encourages adaptive thinking. By continuously exploring and reshaping narratives around trauma, you can shift from a victim mentality to a more empowered perspective. This cognitive restructuring is fundamental in maintaining mental health improvements achieved through EMDR. You can also find another general journaling exercise with prompts to help you reflect on your healing journey.

## Self-Administered EMDR Techniques

We've discussed how EMDR can be practiced with a therapist, but a significant aspect of this strategy is that you can also apply its principles independently. If you don't have access to therapy, you can practice some self-administered EMDR techniques in the following ways:

- **Practice self-administered techniques.** First, let's consider some foundational self-administered techniques using the basic principles of EMDR. These techniques leverage your natural engagement in bilateral stimulation activities such as walking or tapping, which help process unwanted, disturbing thoughts, feelings, and memories (Parnell, 2008). Self-administered EMDR involves using methods that incorporate bilateral stimulation. For example, when experiencing minor stressors, you can employ simple exercises such as the butterfly hug method. This entails crossing your arms over your chest, placing your hands on your shoulders, closing your eyes, and gently tapping your shoulders in an alternating pattern. This practice helps engage both sides of the brain, facilitating the processing of emotions and reducing distress.

- **Explore different accessible exercises.** Specific exercises can be highly beneficial when applying EMDR principles independently. Combining mindfulness practices with bilateral stimulation techniques offers a structured approach to managing emotional triggers. One effective exercise is mindful walking, which includes focusing on each step while consciously engaging in bilateral stimulation through alternating feet. Another example is tactile tapping, where you tap alternately on each side of your body, paired with deep breathing exercises to maintain mindfulness. Creating safe spaces for processing these emotions and practicing these activities is also essential. You can use visualization techniques combined with bilateral tapping to imagine a peaceful place, thus aiding in regulating emotions during stressful times (Compitus, 2020a).

- **Safeguard emotional well-being.** When you're uncovering traumatic events and memories, it's critical to put your emotional well-being first. Establishing clear boundaries ensures that you do not become overwhelmed by your emotions. Recognizing personal limits and developing a heightened awareness of when professional support is necessary is essential. Minor stressors may be manageable through these self-administered techniques, but severe traumas, phobias, and PTSD should always be addressed by a certified clinician (Parnell, 2008). Knowing when to seek professional guidance is a critical aspect of self-care, and seeking this help ensures that your mental health is preserved throughout the healing process.

- **Build a routine.** Building a routine with self-administered EMDR methods influences consistency. It inspires you to integrate these practices into your daily life, improving emotional well-being. Start by setting aside dedicated time each day for these exercises, gradually building them into your routine. Consistency is vital, because regular practice enhances the effectiveness of these techniques.

The benefits of integrating these self-administered EMDR techniques into your daily routine extend beyond immediate emotional relief. Over time, consistent practice promotes enhanced self-awareness, emotional resilience, and a greater capacity to handle stress.

Dedicating time and emotional effort to these exercises will help you create a proactive environment with enhanced mental health and emotional stability. Integrating these techniques into moments of emotional distress empowers you to regain control over your emotions and navigate challenges more effectively.

## *Visualizing for EMDR*

Visualizing can be a great way to recall past experiences and create a safe space for revisiting painful traumas. Here are some prompts that you can follow to envision different scenarios:

1. Imagine a peaceful beach where the waves gently touch the shore. Close your eyes and breathe in the salty air. Visualize yourself walking along the sand, feeling the warmth under your feet. Think about a happy memory on a beach, a family vacation, or a day spent with friends. Let laughter and joy fill your heart. Picture the sun shining and the sound of seagulls in the distance. Embrace the peace of this moment, knowing you are safe and carefree.

2. Consider a time when you faced a challenge. Bring to mind an obstacle you overcame. Visualize the moment just before you took action. See yourself gathering your strength. Picture the people who supported you. Imagine their encouraging smiles and

words. Feel the determination within you grow. When you took that first step, what did you hear? What did you feel? Immerse yourself in that experience and remember the power of your resilience.

3. Think about a place that makes you feel calm. It could be a quiet forest, a cozy corner in your home, or a favorite park. Visualize the sights and sounds around you. Hear the leaves rustling or the birds chirping. Picture the colors and textures that surround you. There may be a soft breeze brushing against your skin. Allow yourself to sink into that space. Know that you can return here whenever you need comfort or peace. Let the feeling of safety wrap around you like a warm blanket.

4. Now, reflect on a meaningful conversation you have had. Visualize the setting where it took place. Were you sitting at a café or perhaps on a park bench? Picture the expressions on each person's face. Remember the words exchanged, and the emotions felt. Visualize the support or wisdom shared. Think about how that conversation made you feel. What insights did you gain? Why was it necessary? Hold onto that feeling of connection and understanding, knowing that such moments enrich your life.

5. Picture a future goal that excites you. Visualize yourself achieving it. What does it look like? Feel the emotions of success as you imagine crossing that finish line or holding that award. Picture the process you took to get there. Visualize every step—the hard work, the late nights, and the effort. Imagine the support of friends and family during this journey. Feel the pride swell in your chest as you see your hard work pay off. Embrace the vision of success and allow it to inspire you.

6. Think about a situation that caused you fear or anxiety. Visualize that moment, but instead of feeling overwhelmed, see yourself facing it with courage. Picture the fear shrinking as you stand firm.

Feel the strength building within you as you confront your worries. Let the feelings of anxiety dissipate. Visualize the support you have from loved ones or counselors. Picture their comforting presence giving you strength. Hold onto this empowerment, knowing you can tackle any challenge that comes your way.

7. Think of a memory that brings you comfort. This could be a childhood moment, a hug from someone you love, or a quiet evening reading. Visualize every detail of that memory: the sounds, smells, and feelings. Picture the warmth that memory brings into your heart. Let it remind you that there are still beautiful moments in life. Allow yourself to fully experience that comfort and realize you can carry that warmth.

8. Think about areas of growth in your life. Visualize the person you wish to become. Picture yourself taking steps toward that version. What new habits are you forming? How do you feel when you get closer to that goal? Imagine the struggles and how you rise above them. Embrace the change you are undergoing.

9. See your support in this journey—the friends and mentors guiding you. Let that feeling of transformation resonate deep within you. Recall a time you felt grateful. Visualize the people, experiences, or things that brought you joy. See their faces and feel the warmth of your appreciation. Imagine the moments that made you smile and laugh. Picture writing a thank-you note to those who impacted your life positively. Let gratitude fill you up and allow this feeling to overflow into your daily life. Remember, gratitude opens the door to more blessings.

10. Imagine your ideal day. What would you do? Visualize the activities you would enjoy and the people you would spend time with. Picture waking up feeling refreshed and excited. See yourself engaging in activities that bring you happiness. It could be

reading a good book, hiking a beautiful trail, or enjoying a delicious meal with friends. Let the joy of this ideal day inspire you. Keep this vision in your mind and strive to incorporate pieces of it into your everyday life.

11. Finally, consider a time when you felt genuinely compassionate. Visualize how that compassion looked and felt. Picture extending kindness to others, whether through words or actions. Imagine the expressions on people's faces as they receive your kindness. Feel the warmth in your heart as you share love and understanding. Allow the experience of compassion to grow within you. Remember that your actions, no matter how small, can create a ripple effect of goodness in the world.

## Journaling Prompts

Journaling can be challenging when you're describing trauma and deep-rooted pain. The following journal prompts can help you navigate sensitive topics with more ease and confidence:

What emotions come up when you think about a painful memory? Write about those feelings without holding back.

Describe a time when you felt truly alone. What thoughts ran through your mind during that moment?

Are there people you wish you could talk to about your pain? Write letters to them, even if you don't send them.

What are some words you associate with your trauma? Explore their meaning and why they resonate with you.

Can you recall a situation that brought you comfort after a difficult time? Describe it in detail.

Write about a safe space you can visualize in your mind. What does it look like, and how does it make you feel?

Is there a particular song, book, or movie reflecting your trauma experience? Write about how it connects to your story.

What do you wish others understood about your struggles? List your thoughts without censure.

Conclude with an invitation to continue processing your thoughts and feelings in a safe and nurturing way.

# Final Thoughts on EMDR

Understanding and applying EMDR techniques offers a pathway to unbelievable emotional healing that you may have never thought possible. This chapter has discussed the core principles of EMDR, showcasing its unique approach to processing traumatic memories and reducing their emotional impact. By engaging in specific eye movements or bilateral stimulation while recalling distressing memories, you can reprocess these experiences and integrate them into a more coherent narrative. This method showcases your brain's innate ability to heal itself, making it a powerful tool for those struggling with anxiety, depression, or other trauma-related conditions.

The structured eight-phase approach of EMDR, along with the use of bilateral stimulation exercises, provides a comprehensive framework for addressing unresolved memories and enhancing emotional regulation. This therapy helps alleviate immediate distress and fosters long-term resilience and cognitive improvements.

As you continue your journey of self-improvement and mental health management, incorporating EMDR techniques can be valuable to your action plan. Whether used alongside other therapies or as a standalone practice, EMDR holds significant promise in promoting holistic emotional healing and overall well-being.

With the last therapeutic approach wrapped up, it's time to discuss some tips and tricks for integrating these various techniques into your daily life.

**Processing tough emotions can feel like a heavy weight, but you don't have to navigate it alone.**

That's why we created this guided journal—to help you work through challenging feelings and practice acceptance using proven ACT techniques. With prompts to explore your emotions, understand triggers, and embrace them without judgment, this journal is a practical way to build emotional resilience and nurture self-compassion.

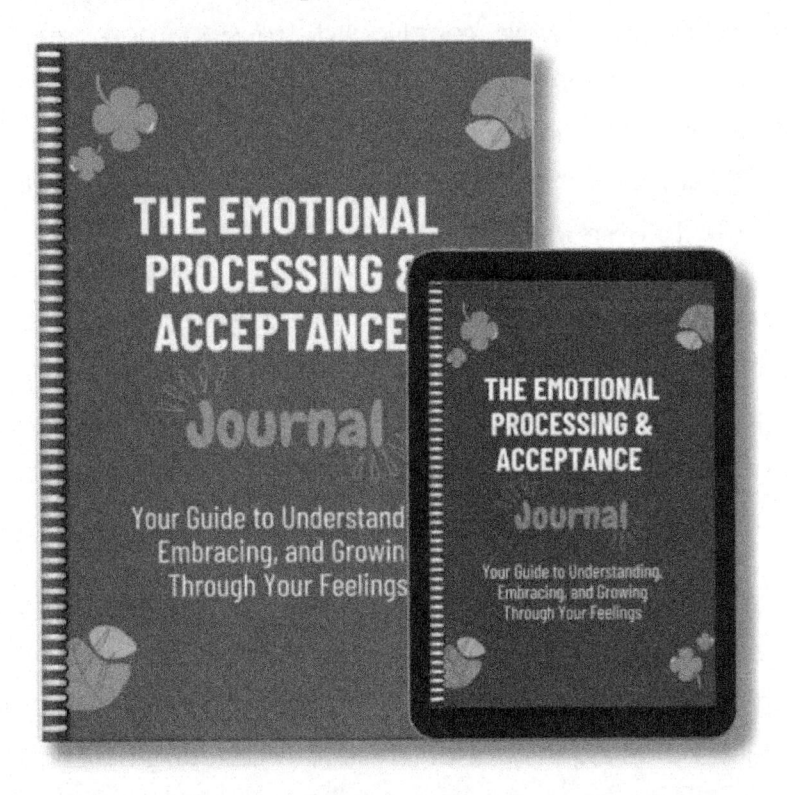

To download your free copy, simply scan the QR Code.
Start your journey toward healing today.

# Chapter 10: Integrative Approaches for Holistic Healing

As you've read through the various practices and techniques throughout this book, you might wonder how you can be expected to choose just one to focus on. The great thing is that you don't have to be limited to just one practice!

Integrative approaches for holistic healing can be achieved by combining various therapeutic techniques to influence emotional, mental, and physical well-being. Each person faces unique emotional and psychological challenges requiring a personalized set of tools. Recognizing the specific areas that need attention can help you select the most effective strategies for your mental health journey. This chapter guides you to identify the challenges that you face through self-reflection. Exploring different therapeutic approaches allows you to develop mental health strategies suited to your needs.

In this chapter, you'll discover how to create a personalized mental health approach by exploring the several therapeutic methodologies discussed throughout this book, including CBT, DBT, and ACT. You will learn how to balance these approaches to create an action plan for holistic healing. You can make relevant decisions for your well-being with practical examples and step-by-step instructions. Whether you're dealing with social anxiety, intense emotions, or chronic pain, this chapter offers actionable steps to craft a mental health action plan that works best for you.

# Creating a Personalized Mental Health Toolkit

Understanding your emotional and psychological challenges helps you find a personalized approach to your mental health issues. We have all had unique experiences, stressors, and triggers that influence our mental health and contribute to the very people that we are today. By identifying specific areas of concern, such as anxiety, depression, or emotional dysregulation, you can select more suitable techniques and strategies that will most effectively address your needs. Here's a deep dive into the strategies you can explore and how you should choose what's best for you:

- **Journal for self-reflection.** Before considering the different therapeutic strategies that you should explore, it's valuable to use your trusted journal as a guide to self-discovery. Self-reflection through journaling or therapy sessions can help uncover these challenges. For instance, someone experiencing high levels of anxiety may benefit from tools focused on stress management and relaxation.

- **CBT.** Once you have a clearer understanding of your emotional landscape, you can explore various therapeutic approaches to find what resonates with you. CBT is an excellent starting point due to its structured approach, which targets the connection between thoughts, feelings, and behaviors. Through CBT, you learn how to identify and challenge negative thought patterns and replace them with more constructive ones. This empowers you to develop healthier coping mechanisms to manage stress and anxiety more effectively (Scheid, 2024).

- **DBT.** DBT offers another set of valuable tools, especially for those dealing with intense emotions or interpersonal issues. It combines cognitive behavioral techniques with mindfulness strategies and teaches you skills in four key areas: mindfulness, distress tolerance, emotional regulation, and interpersonal effectiveness (Scheid, 2024). If you're struggling with emotional regulation, you might find DBT techniques useful in helping you stay present and manage intense feelings without resorting to self-destructive behaviors.

- **ACT.** ACT provides a different angle, encouraging you to accept your thoughts and feelings rather than trying to eliminate them. It focuses on clarifying personal values and committing to actions aligned with those values (Scheid, 2024). This approach helps you create a more fulfilling life while acknowledging the presence of discomfort or negative emotions. If you're dealing with chronic pain, you could benefit from ACT by learning to accept your pain and focusing on doing meaningful activities that are possible despite it.

- **Combine techniques.** Combining techniques from CBT, DBT, and ACT can be particularly beneficial. Integrating different exercises allows for a more comprehensive approach to mental health. For example, using CBT to change negative thought patterns can be complemented by DBT practices to manage emotional responses in stressful situations. Similarly, ACT's emphasis on value- based living can help reinforce the positive changes made through CBT and DBT. This synergy creates a holistic plan to address the multiple facets of your mental health and provides you with well-rounded support. To illustrate this in a real-life setting, consider Megan, an individual who struggles with social anxiety. Megan might use CBT to challenge and reframe the negative thoughts that arise in social situations. Simultaneously, she could apply DBT's mindfulness techniques to stay present and reduce distress during social encounters. Finally, ACT could guide her in focusing on her values, such as building meaningful relationships, which motivates her to engage in social activities despite her anxiety. This multifaceted approach ensures that she has the tools to handle the various aspects of her anxiety comprehensively.

- **Organize your strategies.** Organizing your personalized approach to emotional well-being is crucial to ensure it remains suitable for your needs. Simple organizational strategies can make a significant difference in effectively utilizing these tools. One effective method is to categorize techniques based on the specific challenges they address. For instance, create sections for stress management, emotional regulation, and cognitive restructuring within a journal or a dedicated digital document. This way, when you are faced with a particular issue, you can quickly find the corresponding techniques. Practical examples of organizing your strategy can provide further clarity.

    Consider creating a "mental health binder" where you compile worksheets, journals, and notes on different therapeutic techniques. This binder can have tabs for each type of therapy, making it easy to navigate. Alternatively, digital solutions—apps or online platforms—can serve as interactive toolkits, offering reminders and tracking progress. Apps designed for CBT, DBT, and ACT exercises can be particularly useful, allowing users to access their toolkit anytime and anywhere.

- **Create a weekly plan.** Another helpful strategy is to develop a daily or weekly plan that incorporates different exercises from your action plan. For example, start the day with a mindfulness practice from DBT, followed by a brief CBT exercise to set a positive mindset. Throughout the day, use ACT principles to stay aligned with your values and goals. This structured approach ensures that you consistently engage with various techniques, reinforcing their benefits over time.

To ensure that your approaches always remain relevant to your progress, set aside time for monthly reviews and adjustments. During these reviews, reflect on recent challenges and successes, noting which tools were most helpful. Adjust your strategy plans accordingly by adding new techniques or modifying existing ones. Engaging in this ongoing evaluation ensures that your approaches always remain dynamic and helpful and can continuously support your mental health and well-being.

## Self-Reflection Journal Prompts

To help you identify the strategies and techniques that would work best for you, answering the following journal prompts can be enlightening:

What are my goals for this week? List three specific objectives. Reflect on how achieving these will impact my overall progress. Are there obstacles I anticipate? Write them down and think of possible solutions. How can I stay focused on these goals each day?

What habits do I want to develop? Identify one habit that I can start practicing today. How will this habit contribute to my well-being? Rate my current commitment to this habit on a scale of one to ten. What can I do to increase this score?

Who do I look up to on my personal journey? Write about a person I admire and the qualities they possess.

How can I emulate those qualities in my own life? In what ways have they overcome challenges similar to mine?

What does success mean to me? Describe what achieving my goals would look like. How will I measure my success? What feelings will accompany my achievements? Are there milestones I can set along the way to celebrate small victories?

What are my strengths? List at least five things I believe I am good at. How can I leverage these strengths to face challenges? Are there new skills I would like to develop? Write down any resources I have to help with this growth.

What fears hold me back? Identify one fear that has affected my progress. What steps can I take to challenge this fear? How has it limited my experiences? Rewrite my narrative surrounding this fear.

How do I find motivation? Reflect on what drives me when I face difficult tasks. Is it the end goal, or do I find joy in the process?

Write down a time when I successfully motivated myself. What strategies did I use?

What lessons am I learning? Think about recent experiences, both positive and negative. What insights have they given me about myself? Have I noticed any patterns in my decision-making? How can I apply these lessons to future situations?

How do I handle stress? List my go-to methods for dealing with anxiety. Are these strategies effective? What new techniques can I incorporate to better manage stress? Write down a moment when I successfully navigated a stressful situation.

What does self-care look like for me? Describe my current self-care routine. Is it serving my needs? What new activities could enhance my self-care? Write about a time I neglected self-care and how it affected my overall well-being.

How do I define balance in my life? Considering my various responsibilities, what does a balanced week look like? What areas feel out of balance?

Write down steps I can take to restore equilibrium.

What role does gratitude play in my life? List five things I am thankful for today. How can expressing gratitude improve my mood? Write a note to someone I appreciate and share how they impacted my life.

What have I accomplished so far this year? Reflect on key successes, big or small. How did these accomplishments contribute to my personal growth? What skills did I develop along the way?

How do I practice resilience? Consider a challenging experience from the past. How did I recover from it? Write about the coping strategies I employed. What did I learn that I can apply to future adversities?

Who are my biggest supporters? Write about the role friends and family play in my journey. How do they inspire me?

Are there ways I can show my appreciation for their support?

What do I want to learn next? Identify a skill or subject that intrigues me. Why is it important for my personal development? What resources are available for me to pursue this learning?

How do I manage my time? Reflect on my current time management strategies. Are they effective? What changes can I make to increase productivity? Write about a day when I maximized my time well. What did I do right?

What does community mean to me? Describe how I relate to my community. In what ways do I contribute? Are there opportunities that I have overlooked? Write down one step I can take to engage more meaningfully with my community.

What fears do I have about the future? List any uncertainties that weigh on my mind. How can I challenge these fears? Write about a time when I faced an unknown future and how I coped.

What am I passionate about? Identify activities that make me feel most alive. How can I integrate more of these passions into my life? Reflect on how these passions contribute to my happiness.

What legacy do I want to leave? Consider how I want to be remembered. What values do I want to instill in others? Write down steps I can take to build this legacy today, even in small ways.

How do I celebrate achievements? Reflect on how I typically reward myself for hard work. Are these celebrations meaningful? Brainstorm new ways to recognize my successes moving forward.

What inspires me? List sources of inspiration in my life, such as quotes, books, or people. How can I incorporate more inspiration into my daily routine? Write about how these inspirations motivate me to move forward.

What does my ideal day look like? Describe a day filled with productive and fulfilling activities. How can I create more days like this? Write about any obstacles preventing me from living my ideal day.

How do I deal with failure? Reflect on a recent failure. What went wrong, and what did I learn from it? How can I reframe my mindset around failure as a learning opportunity? Write about someone I know who has turned failure into success.

How will I hold myself accountable? What systems can I put in place to track my progress? Write about a time when accountability led to success for me. What did I learn from that experience?

# Daily Routines for Sustained Emotional Resilience

Daily routines can provide structure, consistency, and emotional support. Establishing effective daily habits can significantly enhance your mental well-being, as well as keep you committed to the turbulent transformative journey ahead. Let's explore some actionable steps and insights to build a routine that is suitable for you and fosters positivity.

### *Establishing Morning Rituals*

Starting the day with positive energy sets the tone for the entire day ahead. A simple morning exercise routine can be incredibly beneficial. Such practices as stretching or a light jog can help wake up your body, improve circulation, and boost your mood by releasing endorphins. Consider incorporating mindful breathing exercises as part of your morning routine. This can be done simply by taking deep, focused breaths to calm your mind, reduce anxiety, and increase present-moment awareness (Hou et al., 2020).

Another valuable morning routine is practicing gratitude. Spend a few minutes each morning reflecting on things that you are grateful for. This simple act shifts your focus from stressors to positives, which can elevate your mood and provide a more optimistic outlook for the day ahead. You can find a gratitude journaling exercise at the end of this chapter.

### *Incorporating Mindfulness Breaks*

Throughout the day, incorporating short, mindful moments can significantly reduce stress and increase focus. Mindfulness doesn't require long sessions; even a few minutes can make a huge difference. For instance, try the "5-4-3-2-1" grounding exercise. Look around and identify five things that you can see, four things you can touch, three things you can hear, two things you can smell, and one thing you can taste. This technique helps refocus the mind and brings you back to the present moment, reducing overwhelming feelings.

Taking periodic breaks to engage in mindfulness activities such as guided meditations or progressive muscle relaxation can also be beneficial. These practices break the monotony of work and refresh your mental energy, thus making you more productive and less stressed.

## Evening Reflection Practices

Ending the day with reflective journaling can consolidate your experiences and emotions throughout the day, which can stimulate a sense of closure. Effective journaling techniques include writing about what went well during the day, the challenges you faced, and how you managed them. Reflect on your emotional responses and identify patterns or triggers that might need addressing.

Setting aside time to write down affirmations or positive statements about yourself can also enhance self-esteem. Keeping a gratitude journal at night, where you list things that you're thankful for from the day, can also reinforce positive thinking and ensure that you end the day on a good note. You'll find a reflection journaling activity at the end of this chapter that you can practice before going to sleep

## Consistency and Adjustment

While establishing routines is crucial, it's equally important to remain flexible and adjust them as needed. Life is dynamic, so your routines should be just as flexible. Regularly revisit and assess your habits. Are they still serving your goals? Are they sustainable? If you find certain routines are no longer effective, don't hesitate to modify them.

## Practical Guidelines for Implementation

If you're on the right track but you're unsure how you can successfully implement these changes into your daily life, consider the following summary of the previous points and use it as a helpful guideline.

### Establishing Morning Rituals

1. Begin your day with light physical activity to boost energy levels.
2. Practice gratitude to foster a positive mindset.
3. Engage in mindful breathing exercises to center yourself.

### Incorporating Mindfulness Break

Utilize short grounding exercises like the "5-4-3-2-1" technique to stay present.

1. Take regular breaks for guided meditation or muscle relaxation.
2. Integrate brief periods of silence and reflection into your busy schedule.

### Evening Reflection Practices

1. Dedicate time for nightly journaling to process your day's events.
2. Write affirmations to reinforce a positive self-image.
3. Maintain a gratitude journal to end the day on a positive note.

### Consistency and Adjustment

1. Regularly review and adjust your routines based on effectiveness and sustainability.
2. Set SMART goals to align your habits with your mental health objectives.
3. Remain open to trying new techniques and adapting as necessary.

Implementing these practical steps requires dedication and persistence. However, the long-term benefits of enhanced structure, consistent positive habits, and emotional resilience make it worthwhile. Remember that the key to success is not perfection but persistence and adaptability in nurturing your mental health through daily routines.

# Building Support Systems and Resources

Of course, life is always easier when you tackle it with friends and family. Building well-rounded support systems is a valuable way to promote your mental well-being and emotional stability. By making use of the valuable forms of support available to you, you can create a more successful journey of healing ahead. Here are some tips that can help you seek support from loved ones so that you can leverage the relationships in your life during this often-overwhelming journey:

- **Support comes in different forms.** It's important to recognize that support can come in different forms. Friends and family often serve as primary sources of emotional support, offering a listening ear, empathy, and encouragement during challenging times. Emotional support may involve conversations where feelings are shared freely, comfort is provided, and a sense of belonging is fostered. Support from people close to you, such as immediate family members or good friends, can include practical help, such as assisting with daily tasks or providing financial aid. It's important to note that effective support doesn't necessarily rely on the number of people but rather on the quality of those relationships (Ozbay et al., 2007).

- **Professional support is always valuable.** If you ever find yourself struggling with the pressure of this journey, seeking professional support is invaluable. Even if you feel mentally and emotionally stable, you can never go wrong with getting extra professional help.

Mental health professionals, such as therapists and counselors, provide expertise through different therapeutic approaches specified to your needs. These professionals offer a safe space to explore issues more deeply so that you can develop effective coping strategies. Seeking professional support can be particularly beneficial when dealing with complex mental health challenges that require specialized knowledge.

- **Relationships require two-way effort.** Building and nurturing these relationships requires effort and intentionality. One effective technique for reaching out to others is to start small by expressing genuine appreciation and interest in their well-being. Simple gestures such as sending a thoughtful message or joining regular social activities can help maintain connections. Consistent communication strengthens your bonds and shows your support system that you are there for them just as much as they're there for you.

- **Turn relationships into safe spaces.** Creating environments where open and honest conversations are encouraged can significantly strengthen relationships. Practicing active listening, where one fully concentrates on the speaker without interrupting, shows respect and validates the other person's feelings. This can lead to deeper mutual understanding and trust. It's important to listen to the people in your life without judgment to make them feel heard and validated.

- **Online connections are just as effective.** Technology has become a powerful tool in maintaining long-distance relationships and keeping us connected through it all. Video calls, social media interactions, and instant messaging allow people to stay connected even despite geographical barriers. Utilizing these tools can keep your relationships vibrant and supportive while contributing positively to your mental health.

- **Use the communal resources you have access to.** Communal resources, such as group therapy sessions and workshops, provide structured environments where individuals can share experiences and learn from one another. Group Therapy offers a sense of solidarity, as participants often face similar challenges and can provide peer support. Workshops conducted by mental health professionals can impart valuable skills and strategies for managing stress, anxiety, and other mental health conditions. Local community resources can also be excellent avenues for finding additional support. Community centers, libraries, and faith-based organizations often host events and programs designed to foster social connections and provide emotional assistance. Engaging with local resources not only provides immediate support but also helps build a broader support network over time.

- **Realize that not all relationships are beneficial.** Unfortunately, not all relationships are beneficial. It is crucial to assess and move away from toxic or unhelpful relationships that may harm your mental well-being. Toxic relationships are characterized by behaviors that consistently undermine, belittle, or manipulate. Such relationships can increase stress and anxiety, making it harder for individuals to focus on their own growth and healing. To identify these harmful connections, you should pay attention to how you feel after interacting with certain people in your life. If feelings of anxiety, guilt, or exhaustion frequently follow these interactions, it might be a sign of a toxic relationship. Setting boundaries is an essential step in protecting yourself. Clearly communicating your limits and expectations can safeguard your mental space and reduce unnecessary stress. In cases where distancing yourself from a toxic relationship isn't straightforward, seeking advice from a trusted friend or mental health professional can provide guidance on how to handle the situation delicately. Building new, healthier relationships can gradually replace the negative impacts of toxic ones.

As you consider all of these tips, it's important to remember that building and maintaining a strong support system is an ongoing process. Relationships evolve and so do personal needs. Regularly evaluate the quality of your support system and make adjustments as necessary to ensure it remains effective. Investing in the relationships in your life creates a well-rounded support network that can be your pillar of strength during challenging times.

## Evaluating Progress and Adjusting Strategies

A regular evaluation of your mental health strategies is crucial for achieving optimal outcomes. This ongoing process ensures that the chosen methods remain effective and allows for necessary adjustments based on evolving needs. Don't forget to journal your progress and make changes as needed. The following real-life examples can illustrate how evaluating your progress reaps optimal results.

Consider the story of Sarah, who initially found relief from anxiety through regular exercise. However, over time, she noticed that her anxiety levels were no longer improving despite her consistent workout routine. After reflecting on her strategies and discussing them with her therapist, Sarah decided to incorporate cognitive behavioral techniques alongside her exercise regimen. This adjustment showed more results than any other strategy she'd ever used in her mental health journey.

Similarly, John's experience emphasizes the power of regular evaluation and adaptation. John struggled with depression and used journaling as his primary coping mechanism. Although journaling helped him initially, he eventually felt it wasn't enough to manage his symptoms. By seeking feedback from his therapist, John learned about the benefits of combining journaling with mindfulness practices. This blended approach allowed him to better manage his depression and improved his overall well-being. Incorporating these lessons into your own mental health strategy requires diligence and openness to change. You can achieve the same results as Sarah and John if you continuously put yourself first each day.

# Long-Term Commitment to Mental Health

A long-term commitment to your mental health journey is essential for achieving an enhanced, happier version of yourself. We should all view our mental health as a lifelong process of growth and learning because that's exactly what it is. By adopting this mindset, you can transform challenges into opportunities for personal development, which is a life-changing mindset shift. These are some ways that you can encourage long-term learning and commitment to mental health:

- **Be open to new life lessons.** Life inevitably presents obstacles, whether they are related to our careers, relationships, or personal aspirations. Instead of perceiving these hurdles as setbacks, reframing them as chances to learn and grow can foster resilience. For instance, when faced with stress at work, rather than succumbing to anxiety, you could see it as an opportunity to develop better time management skills or improve problem-solving abilities. By cultivating a mindset that embraces growth, you can better your emotional regulation and reduce feelings of helplessness.

- **Practice daily.** Integrating these practices into daily activities ensures consistency and reinforces new habits. Practical suggestions for blending therapeutic techniques with everyday routines can make significant differences. For example, incorporating mindfulness exercises into your morning routine can set a positive tone for the day ahead. Simple practices such as mindful breathing during commute times or short meditation sessions before bed can seamlessly fit into busy schedules, enhancing overall mental well-being without feeling overwhelmed. Additionally, engaging in physical activities such as yoga or brisk walking can serve dual purposes—promoting physical health and offering mental clarity.

- **Advocate for yourself and others.** Advocacy plays a crucial role in your mental health journey. Sharing success stories not only breaks the stigma associated with mental illness but also inspires others who might be struggling. Personal testimonies about overcoming depression, managing anxiety, or finding balance through holistic practices can greatly impact community perceptions. Speak about your experiences, because it creates a supportive environment where mental health issues are normalized and addressed openly. Being an advocate for mental health requires active participation in spreading awareness and supporting initiatives that promote mental well-being. This can involve participating in local mental health campaigns, volunteering with support groups, or even creating content that educates others about mental health. Encouraging open dialogues within workplaces and communities fosters inclusivity and understanding, thereby helping you build a more empathetic society.

Remember that the journey ahead is nonlinear and never-ending. Although this may sound daunting, it can be freeing to know that you are forever evolving and adapting. Realizing this can help you develop more realistic expectations, instead of assuming it would be a quick fix. Sustainable mental health practices involve regular self-reflection and adjustments. Just as physical health requires consistent exercise and nutrition, mental health demands ongoing attention and care. Regularly revisiting your mental health strategies ensures they remain effective and aligned with your current needs. Using journals or mental health apps is an effective way for you to track and identify the patterns of these changes.

# Evening Reflections

If you choose to practice your reflective journaling exercises in the evening to end off your day mindfully and calmly, here are some informative gratitude prompts that you can follow:

What are three things that made you smile today? Reflect on these moments and how they affected your mood. Consider the small joys that brightened your day, whether it was a friendly conversation or a lovely view.

What challenges did you face, and what did you learn from them? Acknowledge any difficulties and evaluate how you handled them. Recognizing your growth in tough situations helps you appreciate your resilience.

Who is someone you are thankful for? Think about a friend, family member, or even a stranger who impacted your day positively. Write down what they did that made a difference in your life and express your appreciation for them.

What is one achievement you accomplished today, no matter how small?

Celebrate your efforts, whether you completed a task, helped someone, or took time for self-care. Every small victory counts toward your overall happiness.

What is something in your environment that you feel grateful for? It could be the comfort of your home, the beauty of nature, or a cozy blanket. Acknowledging your surroundings helps reinforce your sense of peace.

What lesson did you learn today that you'd like to remember? Think about an experience that taught you something valuable. It could be related to work, relationships, or even something about yourself.

What positive actions did you take today that contributed to your well-being? Reflect on healthy choices, such as drinking enough water, taking a break, or practicing kindness. These decisions shape your day-to-day happiness.

What personal quality are you grateful for? Identify a characteristic within yourself that helped you during the day. It may be your patience, creativity, or ability to empathize with others.

What is something you look forward to tomorrow? Anticipating future joys can bring excitement and motivation. It could be a planned event, a task you enjoy, or simply enjoying a favorite meal.

How did you contribute to the happiness of others today? Think about how your actions positively affected those around you. Celebrate the small interactions that might have lifted someone else's spirits.

What fear did you face today? Acknowledging fears and reflecting on how you managed them can empower you. Each step outside your comfort zone is a step toward growth.

Who gave you a compliment or shared kind words with you today? Reflect on the impact of their words and how they made you feel. Gratitude for others can strengthen relationships and boost your mood.

What is something you accomplished this week that you're proud of? Look back on the past few days and select a highlight. Celebrating your accomplishments fosters a sense of fulfillment.

What habit are you thankful for cultivating in your life? Consider routines you've developed that support your well-being, whether it's journaling, exercising, or connecting with friends. Recognizing the positive impact of these habits encourages their continuation.

What was your favorite moment of relaxation today? Recall a time when you felt truly at ease, whether it was during a bath, watching a favorite show, or simply lying in bed. Recognizing these moments encourages more relaxation efforts in the future.

What beautiful thing did you see today? It may have been a flower, a sunset, or the smile of someone you love. Identifying beauty in your surroundings uplifts your spirit.

What is a funny moment you experienced today? Laughter is a powerful tool for happiness. Reflect on a humorous incident that brought joy and how it lit your mood.

## Concluding Thoughts

As we reach the end of this chapter and this workbook, it's clear that creating a personalized mental health plan requires a thoughtful combination of various therapeutic techniques. By addressing your specific emotional and psychological needs, you can select tools from CBT, DBT, and ACT that resonate with you most. The blend of these methods ensures a thorough approach to managing your personal mental health challenges.

As you set up strategies that work for you, don't forget to organize your specialized approaches by categorizing your techniques and developing daily or weekly plans. Doing this can make these tools easier to access and use effectively. Regularly updating and reviewing your strategies keeps them relevant and adaptable to changing needs. This dynamic process helps you manage current struggles while also preparing you for future challenges and ensuring long-term mental well-being. This commitment to your journey will help you develop routines and a support system that encourages a healthier, more fulfilling life.

# Conclusion

As we conclude this journey, let's revisit some key concepts that have been explored throughout the book. From the foundational principles of cognitive behavioral therapy (CBT), which help you reframe negative thought patterns, to the mindful practices found in acceptance and commitment therapy (ACT), which teach you to embrace your experiences without judgment, as well as the techniques of dialectical behavior therapy (DBT), which allow you to address your mental and emotional health issues through mindfulness and distress tolerances, each therapeutic approach has been a guide, leading you toward emotional resilience and self-growth. These techniques are not just theoretical; they offer practical pathways that can transform how you navigate your internal landscapes.

On the one hand, CBT has shown you that by identifying and challenging irrational thoughts, you can replace them with healthier, more balanced perspectives. This shift in thinking often leads to remarkable changes in your feelings and behaviors, providing a solid foundation for improved mental health. On the other hand, ACT encourages you to accept your thoughts and feelings rather than fighting or feeling overwhelmed by them. You can leave your suppressed emotions in the past. This acceptance allows you to focus on what truly matters in your life and take committed action toward those values. Additionally, DBT helps you regulate overwhelming emotions that can influence mental health issues such as anxiety and depression.

Additionally, we have delved into mindfulness-based approaches that encourage you to stay present and observe your thoughts and emotions without being swept away by them. These practices build your capacity for awareness and intentionality and help you to respond to life's challenges with greater calm and clarity. Somatic techniques, too, have shown their value by connecting your physical experiences with your emotional states, offering another avenue for healing and self-understanding.

It's important to emphasize that these methods are not meant to be isolated techniques but integrated tools that work synergistically. They serve as parts of a comprehensive mental health toolkit, adaptable to individual needs and circumstances. Each chapter has aimed to provide you with actionable steps and exercises, making these concepts readily applicable to your daily life.

Use this workbook as a starting point for continued exploration and growth. Mental health is like a garden that requires ongoing care and attention. Just as a gardener tends to their plants, nurturing them through different seasons, you must also tend to your mental well-being. The seeds planted through CBT, DBT, ACT, mindfulness, and somatic practices need regular watering and sunlight to bloom into a flourishing life filled with awareness and intention.

It's crucial to remember that personal growth and self-discovery are lifelong processes. This book has equipped you with valuable tools, but the real transformation occurs beyond these pages. Embrace every opportunity for growth, whether it comes from reading more about these topics, attending workshops, seeking therapy, or simply reflecting during quiet moments. Each step you take brings you closer to a more balanced and fulfilling life.

Consistency is key in this process. It's not enough to practice these techniques sporadically. Regular application is what leads to lasting change. Consider setting aside dedicated time each week for your mental health practices. Whether it's journaling, practicing mindfulness, engaging in somatic exercises, or even revisiting some of the activities suggested in this book, consistency will cultivate the deep-rooted changes that you desire. Establishing routines can be incredibly beneficial, turning these practices into habits that support your overall well-being.

As you move forward, keep in mind that your journey is uniquely yours. No two paths to mental wellness look the same, and what works for one person might not necessarily work for you. It's vital to personalize these strategies to fit your specific needs, preferences, and life context. Pay attention to what resonates with you and feels most effective. Your mental health toolkit should be as unique as you are, crafted to support your distinct journey.

Use this personalization to foster a deeper connection with yourself. By tailoring these techniques, you honor your individuality, acknowledging that your experiences, strengths, and challenges are yours alone. This personalized approach not only enhances the effectiveness of the practices but also empowers you to take ownership of your mental health.

Your relationship with your mental health is ongoing and dynamic. There will be periods of progress and times of setbacks, both of which are natural parts of the journey. Approach this process with compassion for yourself. Celebrate your successes, no matter how small they may seem, and view setbacks as learning opportunities rather than failures. Every experience is a chance to grow wiser and more resilient.

If you ever feel stuck or overwhelmed, remember that seeking help is a strength, not a weakness. Engage with supportive communities and reach out to mental health professionals or find peer support groups.

These resources can offer guidance, encouragement, and new perspectives, thus reinforcing your path to emotional well- being. In closing, I hope that the insights and tools shared in this book have provided you with a sense of empowerment and hope. May you continue to explore, apply, and refine these practices, nurturing your mental health with patience and dedication.

Remember that you are not alone on this journey. With each step you take, you are building a life of greater emotional resilience, self-awareness, and intentionality.

May your continued exploration lead to profound growth and fulfillment, enriching your life and the lives of those around you.

## Thank You, Dear Reader!

Congratulations on finishing the book! **I'm so proud of you** for taking this important step toward healing and personal growth. There are countless resources out there, and **I'm truly grateful** that you chose mine to be part of your journey.

If you found this book helpful, **I'd love your support** in keeping it visible for others who need it. Leaving a review on Amazon is quick and easy—it's just 2-3 clicks. Simply **scan the code** to share your thoughts and help others discover these tools for their own healing.

**Thank you again for choosing this book,** and I wish you continued success on your journey.

With gratitude,
**Andrew C. Hinkelberg**

### Scan to leave a review:

# Glossary

**Acceptance and commitment therapy (ACT).** A form of psychotherapy that encourages individuals to accept their thoughts and feelings instead of fighting or feeling guilty about them. It teaches mindfulness skills to help clients live in the moment and commit to actions that enrich their lives.

**Behavioral activation.** A therapeutic approach aimed at helping individuals engage more with their environment and activities that bring pleasure or meaning. It is often used to combat feelings of depression or anxiety.

**Cognitive behavioral therapy (CBT).** A type of psychotherapy that helps people understand and change their thoughts and behaviors. It is based on the idea that your thoughts influence your feelings and actions.

**Desensitization.** This occurs when an individual's emotional response to a stimulus decreases over time due to repeated exposure. It can take place in various contexts, such as in response to violence, emotional pain, or even stressful situations.

**Dialectical behavior therapy (DBT).** A form of CBT that aims to help individuals manage their emotions and improve their relationships. It is particularly effective for those who experience intense emotional responses, often associated with borderline personality disorder, but it can benefit others with mental health issues as well.

**Diary cards.** Tools used in therapy to track emotions, thoughts, and behaviors. They help individuals document their feelings over time. This documentation can provide insight into patterns or triggers in their daily lives.

**Distortive thinking**. A way of processing information that leads to skewed perceptions and decisions. Individuals engaging in this pattern often misinterpret events or experiences, which can result in negative outcomes.

**Distress tolerance**. The ability to manage and endure emotional pain or distress without resorting to harmful behaviors. It involves coping strategies that help individuals handle challenging situations more effectively.

**Eye movement desensitization and reprocessing (EMDR)**. A psychotherapy treatment designed to alleviate the distress associated with traumatic memories. It involves recalling distressing events while receiving bilateral sensory input, such as side-to-side eye movements, taps, or sounds.

**Interpersonal effectiveness**. The ability to communicate and interact with others in a way that is both constructive and respectful. It involves understanding your own emotions and the emotions of others, which enhances relationships.

**Mindfulness**. The practice of being fully present in the moment. It involves paying attention to our thoughts, feelings, and surroundings without a sense of negativity but rather acceptance.

**Positive affirmations.** Positive statements that can help you challenge and overcome negative thoughts. They are designed to boost your self-esteem and improve your mindset.

**Post-traumatic stress disorder (PTSD)**. A mental health condition that can occur after experiencing or witnessing a traumatic event. It often involves persistent memories of the event, nightmares, and severe anxiety.

**Somatic therapy**. A holistic approach that focuses on the connection between the body and the mind. It emphasizes the importance of bodily sensations in the healing process.

**Thought records**. A process to help you understand your thoughts and feelings better. By writing them down, you can see patterns in your thinking, which is especially beneficial for tackling automatic negative thinking.

**Vagus nerve**. One of the longest nerves in the body. It runs from the brain through the neck and into the chest and abdomen. It plays a key role in the autonomic nervous system, which controls involuntary bodily functions.

**Vision board**. A tool that helps people visualize their goals and dreams. It is usually a collage of images, words, and phrases that represent what a person wants to achieve in life.

**Visualization**. The process of creating a mental image or concept of something. It allows individuals to see and understand ideas, feelings, and experiences without needing a physical representation.

# References

Ackerman, C. (2017, March 20). *25 CBT techniques and worksheets for cognitive behavioral therapy.* PositivePsychology.com. https://positivepsychology.com/cbt-cognitive-behavioral-therapy-techniques- worksheets/

Ackerman, C. (2018, February 12). *CBT's cognitive restructuring (CR) for tackling cognitive distortions.* Positive Psychology. https://positivepsychology.com/cbt- cognitive-restructuring-cognitive-distortions/

Ackerman, C. E. (2018, February 5). *21 emotion regulation worksheets & strategies.* Positive Psychology. https://positivepsychology.com/emotion-regulation- worksheets-strategies-dbt-skills/

Ackerman, C. (2017, September 29). *Cognitive distortions: When your brain lies to you.* Positive Psychology. https://positivepsychology.com/cognitive-distortions/

Ala'ilima, K. (2023, July 21). *Bilateral stimulation: What it is, effects, & use in EMDR.* Choosing Therapy. https://www.choosingtherapy.com/bilateral-stimulation/

Altman, D. (2024). *Journaling about trauma: Writing to heal.* Choosing Therapy. https://www.choosingtherapy.com/journaling-about-trauma/

Assaz, D. A., Tyndall, I., Oshiro, C. K. B., & Roche, B. (2022). *A process-based analysis of cognitive defusion in acceptance and commitment therapy. Behavior Therapy, 54*(4), 678-691. https://doi.org/10.1016/j.beth.2022.06.003

Bay. (2024, September 6). *Elevate your mindset with cognitive defusion techniques.* Bay Area CBT Center. https://bayareacbtcenter.com/cognitive-defusion-techniques/

Bay. (2023, August 6). *Vagal toning for anxiety and stress relief.* Bay Area CBT Center. https://bayareacbtcenter.com/vagal-toning-for-anxiety-and-stress-relief/

Beck, J. S., & Fleming, S. (2021, June 18). *A brief history of Aaron T. Beck, MD, and cognitive behavior therapy.* Clinical Psychology in Europe. https://cpe.psychopen.eu/index.php/cpe/article/view/6701

Beck, A. T. (2019, January). *A 60-year evolution of cognitive theory and therapy.* perspectives on psychological science. https://journals.sagepub.com/doi/10.1177/1745691618804187

Beck, A. T., Grant, P., Inverso, E., Brinen, A., & Perivoliotis, D. (2020). Recovery-oriented cognitive therapy for serious mental health conditions. New York, NY, USA: Guilford Press.

Bennett, T. (2023, September 24). *The art of mindful movement: Exploring yoga, Tai Chi, and Qi Gong for holistic health.* Eastside Ideal Health. https://www.eastsideidealhealth.com/the-art-of-mindful-movement-exploring-yoga-tai-chi-and-qi-gong-for-holistic-health/

Betterup. (n.d.). *75 shadow work prompts for healing, growth, & mental health.* https://www.betterup.com/blog/shadow-work-prompts

Breit, S., Kupferberg, A., Rogler, G., & Hasler, G. (2018, March 13). *Vagus nerve as modulator of the brain–gut axis in psychiatric and inflammatory disorders.* Frontiers in Psychiatry. https://www.frontiersin.org/journals/psychiatry/articles/10.3389/fpsyt.2018.00044/full

Carr, B. (2013, April 11). *Live your core values: 10-Minute exercise to increase your success 1.* TapRooT® Root Cause Analysis. https://taproot.com/live-your-core-values-exercise-to-increase-your-success/

*CBT vs DBT vs ACT: What are the types of therapy available.* (2023). Counseling and Wellness Center of Pittsburgh. https://counselingwellnesspgh.com/cbt-vs-dbt-vs- act-what-are-the-types-of-therapy-available/

Chapman, A. L. (2006, September). *Dialectical behavior therapy: Current indications and unique elements.* Psychiatry (Edgmont); Matrix Medical Communications. https://www.ncbi.nlm.nih.gov/pmc/articles/PMC2963469/

Charlie Health Editorial Team (2023, October 27). *CBT journaling can help you deal with negative thoughts.* Charlie Health. https://www.charliehealth.com/post/cbt- journaling

Cleveland Clinic. (2023, June 9). *Exposure therapy.* Cleveland Clinic. https://my.clevelandclinic.org/health/treatments/25067-exposure-therapy

Cleveland Clinic. (2022, November 10). *Relax your way to better sleep (and more).* Cleveland Clinic. https://health.clevelandclinic.org/progressive-muscle- relaxation-pmr

*Cognitive defusion techniques and exercises.* (n.d.). Cognitive Behavioral Therapy Los Angeles. https://cogbtherapy.com/cbt-blog/cognitive-defusion-techniques-and- exercises

Compitus, K. (2020a, July 15). *Your ultimate EMDR therapy guide.* Positive Psychology. https://positivepsychology.com/emdr-therapy/

Compitus, K. (2020b, October 20). *12 radical acceptance worksheets for your DBT sessions.* Positive Psychology. https://positivepsychology.com/radical- acceptance-worksheets/

Cronkleton, E., & Walters, O. (2022, March 16). *Alternate nostril breathing: Benefits, how to, and more.* Healthline. https://www.healthline.com/health/alternate- nostril-breathing

Damasio, A., & Carvalho, G. (2013). The nature of feelings: Evolutionary and neurobiological origins. *Nature Reviews Neuroscience* 14, 143–

152.

*DBT distress tolerance skills (Worksheet).* (n.d.). Therapist Aid. https://www.therapistaid.com/therapy-worksheet/dbt-distress-tolerance-skills

*DBT skills interpersonal effectiveness.* (2023, February 17). Rethinking Residency. https://rethinkingresidency.com/wellness-resources/dbt-skills/dbt-skills-for- increasing-interpersonal-effectiveness/

*DBT: Wise mind - skills, worksheets, videos, & activities.* (n.d.). DBT. https://dialecticalbehaviortherapy.com/mindfulness/wise-mind/

De Young, K. P., Lavender, J. M., Washington, L. A., Looby, A., & Anderson, D. A. (2010). A controlled comparison of the word repeating technique with a word association task. *Journal of Behavior Therapy and Experimental Psychiatry, 41(4), 426-432.* https://doi.org/10.1016/j.jbtep.2010.04.006

*Diary Cards.* (n.d.). DBT Self Help. https://dbtselfhelp.com/diary-cards/

Eeles, J., & Walker, D. (2022, July 8). *Mindfulness as taught in dialectical behaviour therapy: A scoping review.* Clinical Psychology & Psychotherapy. https://doi.org/10.1002/cpp.2764

*Enhancing emotional resilience with cognitive behavior therapy coping skills.* (2024). Grouporttherapy.com. https://www.grouporttherapy.com/blog/cbt-coping- skills?5d78fb30_page=5

Everhealth. *(2024). 5 mindfulness exercises for daily life - Enhance your mental well-being.* Everhealth.net. https://everhealth.net/resources/education/mindfulness- exercise-daily-life

*Exploring the 8 phases of EMDR* (2024). Apa.org. https://www.apa.org/topics/psychotherapy/emdr-phases

Fassbinder, E., Schweiger, U., Martius, D., Brand-de Wilde, O., & Arntz, A.

(2016, September 14). *Emotion regulation in schema therapy and dialectical behavior therapy.* Frontiers in Psychology. https://www.frontiersin.org/journals/psychology/articles/10.3389/fpsyg.2016.0 1373/full

*Five steps to identify your values.* (n.d.). The Leadership Coaching Lab. https://www.theleadershipcoachinglab.com/blog/identify-your-core-values

*Free downloads 2 - CBT worksheets.* (n.d.). Getselfhelp.co.uk. https://www.getselfhelp.co.uk/free-downloads-2-cbt-worksheets/

Fuchs, C., Lee, J. K., Roemer, L., & Orsillo, S. M. (2013, February). *Using mindfulness- and acceptance-based treatments with clients from nondominant cultural and/or marginalized backgrounds: Clinical considerations, meta-analysis findings, and introduction to the special series.* Cognitive and Behavioral Practice. https://www.sciencedirect.com/science/article/abs/pii/S107772291 2000041?via %3Dihub

Godreau, J. (2024, August 9). *24 ways to transform negative thoughts with cognitive behavioral techniques.* Mindful Health Solutions. https://mindfulhealthsolutions.com/24-ways-to-transform-negative-thoughts- with-cognitive-behavioral-techniques/

Harmony, B. (2021, June 6). *Finding calm and self-care: 15 ways to stimulate the vagus nerve at home.* Brain Harmony. https://www.brainharmony.com/blog/2021/6/5/15-ways-to-create-vagal- regulation-at-home

Health, E. B. (2023, December 12). *Mental health goals: Strategies for success in the new year.* Embark Behavioral Health. https://www.embarkbh.com/blog/mental- health/mental-health-goals/

Health, M. (2023, May 16). *7 DBT mindfulness exercises to help control your emotions.* Mental Health Center Kids. https://mentalhealthcenterkids.com/blogs/articles/dbt-mindfulness-exercises

Health, R. (2024, January 29). *Mastering mindfulness: The 5, 4, 3, 2, 1 method for anxiety relief.* Resony Health. https://resony.health/blog/mastering- mindfulness-the-5-4-3-2-1-method-for-anxiety-relief

Herndon, J. (2021, June 10). *Exposure therapy for anxiety: What to expect and effectiveness.* Healthline. https://www.healthline.com/health/anxiety/exposure- therapy-for-anxiety

Hou, W. K., Lai, F. T., Ben-Ezra, M., & Goodwin, R. (2020, July 28). *Regularizing daily routines for mental health during and after the COVID-19 pandemic.* Journal of Global Health. https://jogh.org/documents/issue202002/jogh-10-020315.pdf

*How to stimulate the vagus nerve.* (n.d.). Oxygen Advantage. https://oxygenadvantage.com/science/vagus-nerve-stimulation/

Kashdan, T. B., & Rottenberg, J. (2010, November). *Psychological flexibility as a fundamental aspect of health.* Clinical Psychology Review. https://linkinghub.elsevier.com/retrieve/pii/S0272735810000413

Kaufman, S. (2021, August 13). T*he eight phases of EMDR therapy.* EMDR International Association. https://www.emdria.org/blog/the-eight-phases-of-emdr-therapy/

Keng, S. L., Smoski, M. J., & Robins, C. J. (2011, May 13). *Effects of mindfulness on psychological health: A review of empirical studies.* Clinical Psychology Review. https://www.sciencedirect.com/science/article/abs/pii/S027273581100081X?vi a%3Dihub

Klussman, K., Curtin, N., Langer, J., & Nichols, A. L. (2022, February 25). *The importance of awareness, acceptance, and alignment with the*

self: *A framework for understanding self-connection*. Europe's Journal of Psychology.
https://ejop.psychopen.eu/index.php/ejop/article/view/3707

Kuo, J. R., Fitzpatrick, S., Ip, J., & Uliaszek, A. (2022, May 18). *The who and what of validation: an experimental examination of validation and invalidation of specific emotions and the moderating effect of emotion dysregulation*. Borderline Personality Disorder and Emotion Dysregulation.
https://bpded.biomedcentral.com/articles/10.1186/s40479-022-00185-x

Linehan, M. M., & Wilks, C. R. (2015, April). *The Course and evolution of dialectical behavior therapy*. American Journal of Psychotherapy.
https://psychiatryonline.org/doi/10.1176/appi.psychotherapy.2015.69.2.97

Li, T. W., Liang, L., Ho, P. L., Fung Yeung, E. T., Hobfoll, S. E., & Hou, W. K. (2022, May). *Coping resources mediate the prospective associations between disrupted daily routines and persistent psychiatric symptoms: A population-based cohort study*. Journal of Psychiatric Research.
https://www.sciencedirect.com/science/article/pii/S0022395622002862?via%3Dihub

Li, Z., Shang, W., Wang, C., Yang, K., & Guo, J. (2022, November 14). *Characteristics and trends in acceptance and commitment therapy research: A bibliometric analysis*.
https://www.frontiersin.org/journals/psychology/articles/10.3389/fpsyg.2022.9 80848/full

LMHC, M.-B. Z., M. Ed. (2021, November 30). *3 simple EMDR exercises to practice any time of the day*. EMDR Healing.
https://emdrhealing.com/3-simple-emdr- exercises/

M. M. (2023, July 18). *Cognitive therapy techniques & worksheets: Your ultimate toolkit*. Positive Psychology.
https://positivepsychology.com/cognitive-therapy- techniques/

Mayo Clinic Staff. (2020, September 15). *Mindfulness exercises*. Mayo

Clinic. https://www.mayoclinic.org/healthy-lifestyle/consumer-health/in- depth/mindfulness-exercises/art-20046356

McCallie, M. S., Blum, C. M., & Hood, C. J. (2006). Progressive muscle relaxation. Journal of Human Behavior in the Social Environment, 13(3), 51–66.

Mental Health First Aid. (2020, August 6). *The Importance of having a support system*. Mental Health First Aid. https://www.mentalhealthfirstaid.org/2020/08/the- importance-of-having-a-support-system/

Mongelli, F., Georgakopoulos, P., & Pato, M. T. (2020). *Challenges and opportunities to meet the mental health needs of underserved and disenfranchised populations in the United States.* Focus. https://psychiatryonline.org/doi/10.1176/appi.focus.20190028

Moore, C. (2019, June 14). *21 ACT worksheets and ways to apply acceptance & commitment therapy.* Positive Psychology. https://positivepsychology.com/act- worksheets/

Nash, J. (2022, January 14). *ACT techniques: 14 interventions & activities for your sessions.* Positive Psychology. https://positivepsychology.com/act-techniques/

Nash, J. (2022, January 21). *24 best self-soothing techniques and strategies for adults.* Positive Psychology. https://positivepsychology.com/self-soothing/

Nortje, A. (2020, July 1). *10+ best grounding techniques and exercises to strengthen your mindfulness practice today.* Positive Psychology. https://positivepsychology.com/grounding-techniques/

Ozbay, F., Johnson, D. C., Dimoulas, E., Morgan, C. A., Charney, D., & Southwick, S. (2007, May). *Social support and resilience to stress: From Neurobiology to clinical practice.* Psychiatry (Edgmont); Matrix Medical Communications. https://www.ncbi.nlm.nih.gov/pmc/articles/PMC2921311/

Parnell, L. (2008). *Tapping In: A Step-by-Step Guide to Activating Your Healing Resources Through Bilateral Stimulation.* Sounds True

Adult.

Pietrangelo, A. (2019, December 12). *9 CBT techniques for better mental health.*
    Healthline. https://www.healthline.com/health/cbt-techniques

Porges, S. W. (2021, June). *Polyvagal theory: A biobehavioral journey to sociality.* Comprehensive Psychoneuroendocrinology. https://www.sciencedirect.com/science/article/pii/S2666497621000436?via%3Dihub

Porges, S. (2009). *The polyvagal theory: New insights into adaptive reactions of the autonomic nervous system.* Cleveland Clinic Journal of Medicine. https://www.ccjm.org/content/76/4_suppl_2/S86

Price, C. J., & Hooven, C. (2018, May 28). *Interoceptive awareness skills for emotion regulation: Theory and approach of mindful awareness in body-oriented therapy (MABT).* https://www.frontiersin.org/journals/psychology/articles/10.3389/fpsyg.2018.0 0798/full

*Progressive muscle relaxation: Benefits, techniques, and more.* (2021, August 9). Medical News Today. https://www.medicalnewstoday.com/articles/progressive- muscle-relaxation-pmr

Psychology Tools. (2018). *Using behavioral activation to overcome depression.* Psychology Tools. https://www.psychologytools.com/self-help/behavioral- activation/

Ramirez-Duran, D. (2020, November 11). *Somatic experiencing: Healing trauma with body-mind therapy.* Positive Psychology. https://positivepsychology.com/somatic-experiencing/

Rhandava, I (2024). Personalized strategies for enhancing emotional balance. Coachingly. https://www.coachingly.ai/blog/single/personalized-strategies-for-enhancing-emotional-balance

Roberts, A. E., Davenport, T. A., Wong, T., Moon, H.-W., Hickie, I. B., & LaMonica, H. M. (2021, April). *Evaluating the quality and safety of health-related apps and e- tools: Adapting the mobile app rating scale and developing a quality assurance protocol.* Internet Interventions. https://www.sciencedirect.com/science/article/pii/S2214782921000191?via%3Dihub

Sani, N. A., Yusoff, S. S. M., Norhayati, M. N., & Zainudin, A. M. (2023, February 5). *Tai Chi exercise for mental and physical well-being in patients with depressive symptoms: A systematic review and meta-analysis.* International Journal of Environmental Research and Public Health. https://www.mdpi.com/1660- 4601/20/4/2828

Saunders, N. (2023, April 2). *Breathing techniques to tone the vagus nerve: A simple guide.* Therapy Charlotte. https://www.therapycharlotte.com/breathing- techniques-to-tone-the-vagus-nerve-a-simple-guide/

Scheid, S. (2024, May 15). *Understanding different therapy approaches: CBT, DBT, Mindfulness, and ACT.* Peaks Counseling. https://www.peakscounseling.com/understanding-different-therapy-approaches-cbt-dbt-mindfulness-and-act/

Schmitt, C. M., & Schoen, S. (2022, June 9). *Interoception: A multi-sensory foundation of participation in daily life.* Frontiers in Neuroscience. https://www.frontiersin.org/journals/neuroscience/articles/10.3389/fnins.2022.875200/full

Selva, J. (2018, April 23). *Values clarification: How reflection on core values is used in CBT.* Positive Psychology. https://positivepsychology.com/values-clarification/

SEP, R. K., LCSW, & Claire. (2023, February 3). *5 somatic experiencing techniques that anyone can use to stay grounded.* Life Care

Wellness. https://life-care-wellness.com/5-somatic-experiencing-techniques-that-anyone-can-use-to-stay-grounded/

*Setting goals guide.* (n.d.). Web.sas.upenn.edu. https://web.sas.upenn.edu/sas-hr/goals/

Shapiro, F. (2014). *The role of eye movement desensitization and reprocessing (EMDR) therapy in medicine: Addressing the psychological and physical symptoms stemming from adverse life experience.* The Permanente Journal; National Library of Medicine. https://www.thepermanentejournal.org/doi/10.7812/TPP/13-098

Siegel-Acevedo, D. (2021, July 1). Writing can help us heal from trauma. *Harvard Business Review.*

Spencer-Thomas, S. (2023, May 24). *6 tips to improve your heart rate variability (HRV), Vagal tone, and stress management.* Sally Spencer Thomas. https://www.sallyspencerthomas.com/dr-sally-speaks-blog/2023/5/24/6-tips-to-improve-your-heart-rate-variability-hrv-vagal-tone-and-stress-management

Stepp, S. D., Epler, A. J., Jahng, S., & Trull, T. J. (2008, December). *The effect of dialectical behavior therapy skills use on borderline personality disorder features.* Journal of Personality Disorders. https://guilfordjournals.com/doi/10.1521/pedi.2008.22.6.549

Sunrisertc. (2017a, August 18). *4 steps to happy relationships.* Sunrise Residential Treatment Center. https://sunrisertc.com/interpersonal-effectiveness/

Sunrisertc. (2017b, September 13). *6 life changing skills to successfully manage your next emotional crisis.* Sunrise Residential Treatment Center. https://sunrisertc.com/distress-tolerance-skills/

Sutton, J. (2020, December 16). *Thought records in CBT: 7 examples and templates.* Positive Psychology.com. https://positivepsychology.com/thought-records/

*Survive a crisis situation with DBT distress tolerance skills.* (2019, August 26). Skyland Trail. https://www.skylandtrail.org/survive-a-crisis-situation-with-dbt-distress- tolerance-skills/

Swainston, J. (2021, April 6). *15 behavioral activation worksheets for depression and anxiety.* Positive Psychology. https://positivepsychology.com/behavioral- activation-worksheets/

Therapist Aid. (n.d). *Cognitive restructuring: Socratic questions (Worksheet).* https://www.therapistaid.com/therapy-worksheet/socratic-questioning

Therapist Aid. (2012). *Cognitive distortions (Worksheet).* https://www.therapistaid.com/therapy-worksheet/cognitive-distortions

Tindle, R., Hemi, A., & Moustafa, A. A. (2022, May 23). *Social support, psychological flexibility and coping mediate the association between COVID-19 related stress exposure and psychological distress.* Scientific Reports. https://www.nature.com/articles/s41598-022-12262-w

*Vagus Nerve.* (n.d.). Physiopedia. https://www.physio-pedia.com/Vagus_Nerve

Vereecken, S., Corso, G. (2024, April 22). *Revisiting eye movement desensitization and reprocessing therapy for post-traumatic stressdisorder: A systematic review and discussion of the American Psychological Association's 2017 Recommendations.* Cureus. https://www.cureus.com/articles/247185-revisiting-eye-movement- desensitization-and-reprocessing-therapy-for-post-traumatic-stress-disorder-a- systematic-review-and-discussion-of-the-american-psychological-associations- 2017-recommendations#!/

Websupport_55is7jle. (2024). *The importance of setting SMART goals for success.* Be More Awesome. https://www.bemoreawesome.com/?p=3247

*Why is a diary card an important part of dialectical behavior therapy (DBT).* (2023, June 7). Kairos Wellness Collective.

https://www.kairoswellnesscollective.com/blog/why-is-a-diary-card-an- important-part-of-dialectical-behavior-therapy-dbt

Wilding, C. (2015). *Cognitive Behavioural Therapy*. Hachette.

Wright, K. W. (2023, May 4). Reflective journal: Inspiration, ideas, and prompts. *Day One | Your Journal for Life*. https://dayoneapp.com/blog/reflective-journal/

Wu, A., Roemer, E. C., Kent, K. B., Ballard, D. W., & Goetzel, R. Z. (2021). Organizational best practices supporting mental health in the workplace. *Journal of occupational and environmental medicine, 63*(12), e925-e931.

Printed in Great Britain
by Amazon